The Toxic Consumer

The TOXIC Consumer

L   IN
A F   RLD

Ka   Green
                      .D.,
                      re

STERLING

New York / London
www.sterlingpublishing.com

Printed on recycled paper

STERLING and the distinctive Sterling logo are registered trademarks of Sterling Publishing Co., Inc.

Library of Congress Cataloging-in-Publication Data

Ashton, Karen.
The toxic consumer : living healthy in a hazardous world / Karen Ashton and Elizabeth Salter Green ; foreword by Theo Colborn.
    p. cm. -- (Green essentials series)
  ISBN-13: 978-1-4027-4891-2
  ISBN-10: 1-4027-4891-4
  1. Environmental toxicology--Popular works. 2. Environmental health--Popular works. I. Green, Elizabeth Salter. II. Title.

RA1226.A84 2008
613--dc22

                                   2007034341

10 9 8 7 6 5 4 3 2 1

Published 2008 by Sterling Publishing Co., Inc.
Editorial changes in the American edition
© 2008 by Sterling Publishing Co., Inc.
387 Park Avenue South, New York, NY 10016
Previously published in Great Britain
in 2006 by Impact Publishing Ltd
12 Pierrepont Street, Bath, BA1 1LA
© 2006 by Elizabeth Salter Green and Karen Ashton
Distributed in Canada by Sterling Publishing
c/o Canadian Manda Group, 165 Dufferin Street
Toronto, Ontario, Canada M6K 3H6
Distributed in Australia by Capricorn Link (Australia) Pty. Ltd.
P.O. Box 704, Windsor, NSW 2756, Australia

Book design and layout: Amy Henderson

Manufactured in the United States of America
All rights reserved

Sterling ISBN-13: 978-1-4027-4891-2
      ISBN-10: 1-4027-4891-4

For information about custom editions, special sales, premium and corporate purchases, please contact Sterling Special Sales Department at 800-805-5489 or specialsales@sterlingpublishing.com.

For Florence, Frederick, and Ava May

Thank you to WWF-UK for their groundbreaking work
in the area of toxic chemicals

Contents

CHAPTER 6
Hope and Risks for the Future 128

Foreword

As I think back almost sixty years to when I was expecting my first child, I am constantly reminded how lucky I was. A pregnant woman's worry in the 1950s focused on what color to paint the nursery and what the baby's name would be. In those days we were told that there were placental and blood-brain barriers that protected our developing child from anything the mother might ingest or inhale during her pregnancy. Both my husband and I were pharmacists and like everyone in the medical profession, we believed this. As soon as our babies were born we counted their toes and fingers and when we found ten of each we relaxed and gave thanks. It was all so simple. Little did we know how that would change over the next three generations.

Society in the 1950s was ready to put memories of the Depression and World War II behind it and to move into a more secure and enlightened era. The major corporations that had pitched in to help win the war rapidly converted their technology to make the world a safer and more comfortable place to live. They took advantage of the rapid advances in chemical and engineering technology that grew out of the war and started producing life-saving "wonder-drug" pharmaceuticals, crop-protecting pesticides, and innumerable industrial plastics and fire retardants that created a utopian and euphoric period in modern history. As their sales soared they joined forces with the growing public-relations industry and inculcated a sense of trust in the public about the safety of the chemicals beginning to accumulate in our bodies. Advertisements read like fairy tales—"Better living through chemistry" and "Plastics make it possible" —while at the same time spoon-feeding consumerism to a rapidly growing population.

Very few people knew that the new chemicals were made from the by-products of cracking crude oil to make gasoline and the processing of natural gas to heat our homes. Indeed, it was a brilliant and extremely profitable strategy to get rid of the endless volumes of fossil fuel wastes. These new-age chemicals also made it possible to transport electricity to the most remote regions on earth; to produce high-speed automobiles and airplanes, converting us to a mobile society almost overnight; and to turn vast, diverse farmland acreage into monocultures "to feed the world."

As industry designed chemicals to make our lives better (and their profit margins greater), they failed to create tests to detect their effects in the environment or to ascertain what they would do to us or to our babies in the womb. In the meantime the chemicals were gradually invading every aquatic and terrestrial system in the world. It took us another forty years, until 1990, to finally face up to the reality that the same chemicals that had purported to improve our lives were also undermining the very fabric of what makes it possible for animals and humans to reproduce. It was almost impossible to perceive that many of the chemicals that had become an integral part of our lifestyle and economy could threaten the longevity and integrity of species, as confirmed by obvious damage among wildlife. It makes one ask "How could this happen?"

Quite simply, toxicology failed miserably to detect chemicals that can alter the destiny of our children even before they are born. Toxicological testing protocols were based on the ancient paradigm that "the dose makes the poison." That dogma, like saying "toxic chemicals are only dangerous in high doses," has now been shown to be only half true. Unfortunately, toxicological tests were not designed to determine the safety of factory-made chemicals in the womb. They did not take into consideration that the developing embryo is dependent upon infinitesimally small concentrations of hormones and auxiliary chemicals and the slightest shift in their concentrations in the womb environment can alter how the baby develops and functions throughout its life. Although all life is continually under the control of the endocrine system, we now know with certainty that it is the earliest life stages that are the most vulnerable and that timing of exposure is as critical as the dose.

I can only begin to perceive the dilemma young couples face today as they begin to start a family. Selecting nursery colors and offspring's names are trivial compared to the decisions they will make every day as they decide where to live, where to shop for food, and which products to bring home. The twenty-first-century mother needs to know how to prevent toxic chemicals from getting into her womb and interfering with natural chemicals that control how her baby will develop. The answer of course is to develop awareness of one's surroundings and become knowledgeable about endocrine-disrupting chemicals.

This book was designed for the twenty-first-century family. It is an easy-to-read handbook that should be passed from one generation to the next. In an ideal world, every woman would read this book in preparation to bear children and also to set an example for her daughters and sons as they reach the age of having children. Most important, twenty-first-century *fathers* must read this book. They often share child-care duties, they have to make purchasing decisions every day, and through their reproductive cells they can have a profound impact on the health of their male progeny through four generations if exposure takes place early in development.

It is important to note that in this modern world, *everyone* at every stage of life needs this book. Exposure to endocrine disruptors at any age, not just in utero or in childhood, has been linked with some of the increasingly prevalent disorders that just three generations ago were considered rare.

This book will sensitize readers so that they instinctively learn to create a cleaner environment and parents so that they pass this habit on to their children. We live in a time where every purchasing decision should take chemical exposure into consideration. Just as our ancestors adapted to one hazard after another, the successful twenty-first-century family must adapt to the hazards posed by widely dispersed endocrine-disrupting chemicals in the environment. This book will help families increase their probability of reproducing and giving birth to healthy, intelligent children with the ability to reach their fullest potential.

Theo Colborn, Ph.D.
President, The Endocrine Disruption Exchange (TEDX)
Professor, University of Florida, Gainesville
co-author of *Our Stolen Future*

Preface

This book seeks to show that there is an increasing body of evidence pointing to a possible link between the rise of certain non-infectious human health problems and the increase in our exposure to many synthetic chemicals. We are unable to state categorically that toxic man-made chemicals are the cause of certain illnesses or are necessarily detrimental to human health, because of the plethora of different factors that affect any given individual at any one time. What we do know for certain is that the widespread use of man-made chemicals in industrialized nations has led to global contamination of the environment, wildlife, and humankind, and that many chemicals in everyday consumer products have been found to contaminate human tissue. The presence of certain man-made chemicals at current environmental levels may well be having a negative impact on both wildlife and human health. The results of laboratory studies, case histories of accidental chemical contamination in the past, the direct measurement of chemical exposure in humans, and correlative data between levels of exposure to chemicals and the incidence of certain disorders—these all support the wisdom of adopting a precautionary approach with regard to hazardous chemicals. This book supports the view that we should minimize our exposure to those chemicals suspected to have toxic effects until the full extent of their toxicity on human health has been determined—and, where chemicals are shown to be toxic to human health, that safer alternatives should be sought.

Introduction

The extent to which man-made chemicals, in their relatively short history, have become infused into the fabric of twenty-first-century lifestyles is astonishing. The first synthetic chemicals were created in the late 1800s, but it wasn't until after World War II that the industry really took off. Chemists previously working on chemical weapons for combat use realized that many of the deadly poisons they had been concocting had a useful peacetime role: to wage agricultural war against the various pests and insects that damage crops. Shortly after that came the realization that other synthesized chemicals of similar structure could be employed, at great profit, to "improve" our consumer products and way of life. Coinciding with postwar prosperity in the developed world and increased demand for luxuries, many of the chemical industry's innovations were focused on making life easier—and so the industry exploded with thousands of novel molecular structures. This from DuPont in the 1950s:

"Better things for better living . . . through chemistry"

. . . thereby heralding the coming of age of nonstick, easy-clean, disposable living. But, as most of us know from experience, there is no such thing as a free lunch. There's nearly always a downside when things come too easily—and this is one part of the story of man-made chemical production at the turn of the twenty-first century. Synthetic chemicals are largely used in consumer products to make things more attractive, easier to use, longer lasting, smoother gliding, and so on. But how enthusiastic would the average consumer be about a product if it also offered a significant dose of toxicity as part of its "new-and-improved" formula?

A growing body of evidence suggests that certain chemicals found in everyday products can compromise fertility and jeopardize the normal development of the fetus in utero. Furthermore, they may be disruptive to neurological function and to the normal processes of the body's own chemical messaging system (the endocrine or hormonal system), and they are implicated in causing cancer. What is more, many of these chemicals are *bioaccumulative*; that is, they build up in our body fat and never leave.

In many ways, the last few decades have been a three-way conspiracy of ignorance between short-sighted, high-profit invention, consumer desire for everything new-and-improved, and extraordinary regulatory laxity. As a result, some sectors of the chemical industry have single-handedly, and with great speed, contaminated all four corners of the world. Toxic man-made chemicals are now an unavoidable global issue. They are found in places far removed from the factories that create them and the consumer societies that use them, often unknowingly. They are in the air we breathe, the water we drink, the food we eat, the very earth under our feet—and they are in us: in our fat, blood, liver, and brain—and even in our newborn babies.

Chemical Dependency

The chemical industry is vast. It employs over ten million people globally, and its products account for about 7% of the world's GNP (the aggregate economic output of all nations combined). It is important to state that we do have a lot to thank this industry for. Many of the things we take for granted in modern life are due to the spectacular innovations of this sector, such as pharmaceuticals, pigments for dyes, monomers to make plastics, and precursors (chemical compounds that lead to other, usually more stable, products). However, since the industry took off in the 1940s and '50s, the number of new chemical compounds that have been introduced has been staggering—well over 80,000 in the last fifty years alone. And new ones continue to be developed at that same breakneck pace. Yet, with minimal—if any—testing for their impact on health and the environment, thousands of these have found their way into homes, consumer products, and the larger environment.

More staggering is the number of these chemicals that are in the products that we use intimately in everyday life: the ones we slather over our skin, wrap our food in, paint on our fingernails, clean our kitchen stoves with, lay on our floors, and put straight into the mouths of our babies. Most extraordinary of all is that the vast majority of these chemicals have never been adequately tested for their safety for humans or the environment. Of the ones that have been tested, few have been subjected to sufficient rigor. For example, a chemical might have been tested for its effect on a healthy, fully grown male, but not for how it could affect the developing fetus.

> **"A growing body of research shows that pesticides and other contaminants are more prevalent in the foods we eat, in our bodies, and in the environment than we thought."**
> —*Consumer Reports* (Feb. 2006)

According to a report in the *Journal of the American Medical Association* (JAMA), cancers not related to smoking have increased significantly in the U.S. over the past several decades. The report concludes that baby boomers have from 30% (women) to 100% (men) more of these cancers than people of their grandparents' generation, and that the likely cause is "changes in carcinogenic hazards."[1] More recent data from the National Cancer Institute's SEER program show that the incidence of new cancers has risen from 400 cases per 100,000 in 1975 to 482 per 100,000 in 2001. While we cannot blame these increases entirely on toxic chemicals, evidence is growing that they, along with other lifestyle factors, play a key role in rising cancer rates. We should be increasingly concerned about these risks and the fact that, as consumers, our exposure to these chemicals is largely involuntary.

Consenting Adults

Most of us do things from time to time that we know can have a negative impact on our health: drinking alcohol, eating saturated fats, or smoking cigarettes, for example. Sometimes we do these things in moderation; sometimes we do them to excessive and dangerous levels. But whatever your vice and however much you indulge it, it is at least a choice that you yourself have made with some awareness of the risks attached.

This book is concerned with toxic chemicals having either proven or strongly implicated effects on our health, but which we are often exposed to without any choice. They are chemicals that we don't even know are there. There is a long list of everyday consumer products that we use frequently that contain an incredible number of synthetic chemicals, the effects of which on our health—short-, medium-, and long-term—are largely unknown. Current research has shown many synthetic chemicals to be toxic and implicated in a range of health issues, including behavioral problems, declining sperm counts, neurological impairment, birth defects, allergies, diabetes, and various cancers.

Furthermore, as well as being everywhere, many toxic chemicals also act promiscuously, leaching out of the product that originally contained them and contaminating the wider environment. They can enter the food chain and are capable of traveling such vast distances on global airstreams that probably not a single species of living thing or a solitary area of this earth remains uncontaminated by man-made chemicals. Think of the pristine vistas of the polar ice caps, visions of seeming purity; incredibly, these arctic regions are now polluted with some of the most toxic chemicals on the planet, as are the people and wildlife that live there.

So, why are we so blissfully, if dangerously, ignorant? Largely because for many decades, the chemical industry was allowed to put products on the market with little or no safety testing. Only when serious problems came to the public's attention through a catastrophic event, a high-profile lawsuit, or a media exposé would action be taken to control or ban the chemical. The burden of proof of safety has not been on the industry producing the chemical—instead, it has fallen to the public to prove that damage has been done. So now we have tens of thousands of inadequately tested chemicals in products, and an ever-growing body of scientific evidence implicating a significant number of them in serious health effects.

Since the harmful consequences of many common toxic chemicals do not become apparent for years, sometimes decades, significant con-tamination has often already occurred and irreversible harm been done before any action is taken. For example, although a group of chemi-cals called PCBs is now banned, we will be living with their toxic legacy for hundreds of years. In the case of DDT, banned in this country in the seventies, all of us probably have it in our blood—even if we were born yesterday.

This is because the effects of some of the most threatening chemi-cals can be long-term, building up in our body fat over years and being transferred to our children in the uterine environment, via breast milk, and through the food chain. Others have more short-term influences; but if exposure happens at a critical time, for example to a pregnant woman, the effects on her unborn child can be profound. It is impor-tant to realize that there are many products that should really carry warnings: "Use this at your own risk! It contains chemicals that have not been properly tested for their short- or long-term effects on humans, wildlife, or the environment. The most recent scientific evi-dence gives us cause for concern." So far, they don't, so it really is up to us to find out for ourselves.

As long ago as 1962, the American biologist Rachel Carson wrote a groundbreaking book named *Silent Spring* (in reference to the season, not the water source). In it, she warned of the dire potential fallout of the previous quarter century's contamination of life on earth by toxic man-made chemicals:

> **"For the first time in the history of the world, every human being is now subjected to contact with dangerous chemicals, from the moment of their conception until death"**

Close to a half century later, her major concerns relating to pesticides and insecticides have proven accurate, and although many of these have now been strictly regulated or banned, they often still persist in the environment. Catastrophic levels of these older, potent chemicals were released recklessly into the environment in modern industrialized nations and given as aid to Africa. They are still poisoning the breast milk of all women, but particularly Inuit women living in the Arctic. This will be explained in the last chapter, which relates to the broader environmental consequences of chemicals. At this stage, it's mentioned to highlight the incredible potency of some man-made chemicals.

Thankfully, due to improved science and the start of better regulation, contamination levels of the older chemicals cited by Rachel Carson are finally dropping. But we should remain mindful of the potential of other new compounds that have a similar chemical structure and thus might have similar effects. Perhaps even more urgently, we need to understand how they might act together in so-called "toxic cocktails." Since *Silent Spring* was published, tens of thousands of new chemicals have been produced with little or no testing for their potential impact on our health or the environment. And since many of the newer chemicals are not as environmentally persistent or bioaccumulative, we might see serious health effects but not know which chemical is responsible, because it has already broken down and left the body.

Fortunately, the tide is now turning and there is a growing awareness of the serious issues relating to many synthetic chemicals. Environmental groups such as WWF, Friends of the Earth, and Greenpeace have worked very hard and had some success in getting these issues taken seriously at the top levels of government and regulatory agencies, despite intense resistance from certain sectors of the chemical industry. One major reason for the environmental groups' success is that it is no longer possible to ignore the results of research and the irrefutable, observable effects of certain synthetic chemicals over time. The time for rigorous testing and tighter control is now, and most developed countries are placing the subject of toxic chemicals— significant environmental pollutants—high on the political agenda, not only nationally but internationally as well.

It is not the intention of this book to criticize the entire chemical industry. It is an industry that has immeasurably improved modern life. But, like all powerful industries, it needs to be adequately regulated. This has not yet happened. It is essential that the general public be aware of the inherent dangers of certain common chemicals and that we know where they are to be found. We do not pretend to have all the answers. Much more research needs to be done before definitive facts can be made widely available to the general public.

What we are saying is that, in the case of synthetic chemicals with suspected toxicity, where we really don't know the full extent of their health effects, we should err on the side of caution. There are enough examples of serious impacts on our health in recent times to make this the only sensible approach. Understanding some straightforward facts about synthetic chemicals, about their widespread use in manufacturing and modern consumer products—and how the toxicity of some can affect our health and well-being—will help individuals make informed choices about what products they buy for use in their homes, cars, workplaces, and schools.

This book will help its readers to become more aware of the extent to which we are all exposed to dangerous chemicals, and it will offer practical alternatives to help minimize exposure, thereby improving health and longevity. Since it is no longer possible to totally avoid harmful chemicals, taking measures to reduce exposure is the only sensible option for individuals, governments, and industry alike. Furthermore, consumers' knowledge and their collective purchasing power can help compel industry to provide us with non-toxic options that are cleaner, greener, and more healthful for all.

CHAPTER 1

What Are Toxic Chemicals and How Are We Exposed?

This book will provide you with a framework to help you understand the hazardous role that everyday toxic chemicals play in contemporary life. We will describe in detail

- the most potentially harmful substances,
- where to find them,
- the main ways we are exposed to them, and
- why these chemicals are such a cause for concern, personally and environmentally.

We will show that, although toxic chemicals are an unavoidable fact of life, simply by knowing what and where they are, you can take action to significantly reduce your exposure. With this knowledge, you can improve the quality of your immediate environment and protect your health and that of your family.

What Are Toxic Chemicals?

WHAT IS TOXIC? In a general sense, an easier question to answer would be: What's not toxic? Even water, if too much of it is consumed at once, can be harmful, potentially fatal. A *toxic substance,* however, is generally any substance that enters the environment in a quantity or concentration that may have an immediate or long-term harmful effect on the environment, or on human or animal health. A *toxin,* on the other hand, refers to a poisonous substance produced in nature by certain plants, animals, or bacteria that can harm or kill other living organisms—like snake venom, bee-sting poison, or botulin. We are not dealing with toxins here.

Toxic chemicals, for the purposes of this book, are *synthetic* (man-made) chemicals, primarily produced out of organic (i.e., carbon-based) chemistry. We are concerned here with chemicals released into the environment in sufficient concentrations to potentially harm humans, animals, or the environment. In some cases, those levels are almost too small to imagine, particularly when considering a chemical's effects on the developing fetus. Naturally occurring toxic chemicals, such as lead and cadmium, can also present serious health risks, but we will only be covering man-made chemicals.

The Cocktail Effect

Determining the toxicity of a chemical can be very difficult. The concentration and length of exposure required to cause harmful effects can vary widely. In fact, it's not possible to assess the toxicity of all possible variations of chemicals working together to create what's called a *cocktail effect.* It may be the case that an individual chemical is shown to be "safe," but exposure to it in combination with one or more other chemicals may produce toxic effects. The reality is that we are never exposed to one chemical at a time. In everyday life, we are exposed to a vast chemical cocktail. *Additive effects* of multiple chemicals are being seen in laboratory experiments, and it is likely that there will be similar effects in humans too. Hence we advocate a policy of caution and recommend minimizing exposure to all chemicals that have been shown to be toxic or potentially so. We believe this is the only sensible course of action for governments and industry as well (see Chapter 5).

> **In everyday life we are never exposed to one chemical at a time; we are exposed to a vast chemical cocktail.**

Food Choices

We are primarily concerned in this book with synthetic chemicals used in the manufacture of common consumer products, from nail polish to cars. We are not dealing with agrochemicals—agricultural pesticides and insecticides. Where we do discuss food, it is in relation to the way it is processed, prepared, and packaged.

CHOOSING HEALTHFUL FOOD

Our baseline advice regarding what you eat is as follows:

- Select as much of your diet as possible from as low down the food chain as possible: plenty of fresh fruit and vegetables.
- Choose organic produce if available.
- Avoid processed food.
- Ensure that any meat or fish you consume is from known, "clean" sources (for example, the Atlantic is generally less polluted than the Mediterranean) and, again, choose organic wherever possible.

Be aware that the food we eat is generally subject to the phenomena of bioaccumulation and *biomagnification* detailed below. Even organic meat and fish, because they are higher up the food chain than vegetables, will contain significant concentrations of common toxic chemicals. We are not advocating vegetarianism, just moderation, balance, and a generally healthful eating regime.

"Organic" Chemicals?

Not to be confused with "organic" foods and products, organic chemicals are simply compounds of hydrogen and carbon synthesized artificially in places like the laboratory. Organic chemistry is the foundation from which modern, man-made chemicals are produced; it has given rise to a vast array of plastics, solvents, flame retardants, preservatives, waterproofers, plasticizers, surfactants, and many other substances used in the production of consumer goods.

Key Traits of Toxic Chemicals

PERSISTENT CHEMICALS are those that don't readily break down in the environment, but rather linger for years, sometimes decades. When chemicals are continually released into the environment and don't break down, their concentration will inevitably increase. If a persistent chemical is also toxic, then widespread contamination and long-term harm can occur (see Chapter 3 on PCBs).

FAT-LOVING MOLECULES are substances that are predominantly *lipophilic* in nature, which literally means lipid-loving or fat-loving. Lipophilic chemicals don't readily dissolve in water, making them hard to metabolize. Once they've entered the body, they tend to remain in the fatty tissues, including the fat content of the blood, brain, and liver.

If a substance is both lipophilic and persistent, then it can be readily taken up by organisms from contaminated environments such as soil and water. From there, it can bioaccumulate in the food chain.

BIOMAGNIFICATION exacerbates the effect of toxic chemicals to an alarming degree. With chemicals that bioaccumulate, every time something higher up the food chain eats something below it that's contaminated, the concentration increases exponentially by a process called biomagnification. By the time it reaches the top of the food chain, the concentration of a persistent, bioaccumulative chemical can be many *millions* of times that of the original environmental contamination. Persistence, toxicity, and bioaccumulation result in a *toxic body burden,* which may lead to a toxic effect, such as acute or chronic illness or developmental abnormality.

PBT CHEMICALS have several of the above traits at once: they are *persistent,* bioaccumulative, and *toxic.*

Persistent Organic Pollutants

POPs (persistent organic pollutants) are chemicals that exhibit, to a dangerous degree, all three criteria of PBTs: persistence, toxicity, and bioaccumulation. POPs are known to be extremely hazardous. Examples include pesticides (e.g., DDT), industrial chemicals (e.g., PCBs), and the by-products of industrial processes (e.g., dioxins and furans). These chemicals now surround us in daily life; we are constantly exposed to them. POPs are capable of traveling through water and air to regions far away from their source and can cross boundaries of geography and generations. The twelve most potent and most dangerous to human (and wildlife) health, known as the "dirty dozen," are already strictly regulated under a United Nations global treaty known as the Stockholm Convention (2001), commonly called the

POPs Convention. Organizations such as the World Wildlife Fund (WWF) believe that many more chemicals with similar characteristics should be added to the list—for example, certain brominated flame retardants (BFRs; see Chapter 3), a chemical group widely used to prevent common consumer products from going up in flames too quickly in the event of fire. Although flame retardants undoubtedly save lives, safer alternatives with side effects that are less toxic are available, and more need to be developed for widespread use.

THE DIRTY DOZEN

1. PCBs	7. Endrin
2. Dioxins	8. Chlordane
3. Furans	9. Hexachlorobenzene (HCB)
4. Aldrin	10. Mirex
5. Dieldrin	11. Toxaphene
6. DDT	12. Heptachlor

These twelve dangerous persistent chemicals are strictly regulated under the Stockholm Convention, a United Nations global treaty.

Endocrine-Disrupting Chemicals

EDCs (endocrine-disrupting chemicals) are chemicals that can interfere with the endocrine or hormonal system, the body's own chemical messaging system. Our hormones regulate bodily functions such as metabolism, sexual development, and growth. Hormones are released into the blood by various glands, including the testicles, ovaries, and thyroid, and include the sex hormones estrogen (female) and testosterone (male). The endocrine system is a finely balanced one, and is profoundly connected to the nervous and immune systems. Since the most minuscule levels of hormone have great effect, endocrine-disrupting chemicals can play havoc with nature—particularly at critical stages of development, and especially during the complex process of development before birth (see Chapter 2). EDCs can have a variety of end points (chemical effects). They can block natural hormone action, mimic it, or have an opposing effect. Chemicals that interfere with sex hormones in this way are sometimes referred to in the popular media as "gender-benders." EDC effects were first seen in wildlife; various experiments have since shown that EDCs found in common consumer products are implicated in both sexual malformations and confused sexual behavior in animals. Similar effects are becoming increasingly evident in humans. There is a growing body of scientific research that suggests a link between certain EDCs and problems with the human reproductive system, including birth defects, sperm count decline, and sexually related cancers.[2]

Leachates

LEACHING refers to the migration of chemicals from products into the environment. The problem is that some chemicals do not stay locked inside the products they are originally added to and can *leach* out during normal everyday use of the product. They can accumulate in house dust, in the air, and in food and can contribute to indoor pollution as well, contaminating the general environment. A chemical that leaches out of a product can be called a *leachate*. Common examples are bisphenol A, a chemical used to line food cans, which can leach into the contents, and certain flame retardants that leach out of the plastic casings of electrical equipment like TVs and computers and into the air.

Volatile Organic Compounds

VOCs (volatile organic compounds) are compounds that have the ability to evaporate or readily vaporize at room temperature. If these compounds are toxic, they will contribute to indoor air pollution and potentially pose a health risk. Paints, cleaning products, glues, PVC flooring, MDF/particleboard, carpeting, and polishes all commonly contain VOCs that may "off-gas" into the environment around them. (*Off-gassing* is the process whereby gaseous pollutants escape into the environment from the objects and products that contain them.) Formaldehyde is one of the most common VOCs in domestic environments (see Chapter 3).

The Toxic Body Burden

We are constantly exposed to chemicals, both naturally occurring substances and synthetic ones, to those that are toxic and those that are not. The term toxic body burden refers to the amount of toxic chemicals that are present in the body at any given time.

Whether and how a chemical enters the body, and how long it stays there, depends on the intrinsic nature of the substance and the degree of exposure. Exposure can vary, depending on the state the chemical is in (liquid, gaseous, or solid), the prevailing environmental conditions, and, in the case of consumer products, how we use them. Some chemicals are readily metabolized (broken down and excreted) by the body. Others that are persistent and bioaccumulative can remain in our tissues for decades. Even easily metabolized chemicals, if we are exposed to them daily, will be a constant factor in our overall toxic body burden. Though the level may vary, each of us has a toxic body burden, whether we live in an urban high-rise or an isolated cabin, by the ocean or next to an industrial plant.

HOW TOXIC CHEMICALS GET INTO US

- **Ingestion**—We regularly eat foods that have been contaminated with toxic chemicals. This may be through bioaccumulation in the food chain, from food production processes, or from packaging materials. However the chemicals get there, fatty foods are more likely to contain bioaccumulative or lipophilic toxic chemicals than non-fatty foods. Toxicity from agrochemicals also affects many, if not most, non-organic fruit and vegetables. Exposure can also occur from drinking contaminated water, milk, and other liquids.

- **Inhalation**—Toxic chemicals can leach out of the products that contain them into the air, creating both indoor and outdoor air pollution.

- **Transdermal**—Some chemicals are absorbed through the skin when using skin-care products, treated fabrics, and other substances or materials that come in contact with our skin.

- **Through the placenta and breast milk**—The developing fetus will necessarily receive some of its mother's toxic body burden through the placenta; after birth, the child will receive more through breast milk. This is an unavoidable reality of living in such chemical times. It is generally accepted that a mother will pass on approximately 30% of her own toxic body burden to her first-born child. We do not advise against breast-feeding: It is the best possible start for a baby, providing the perfect balance of nutrients and immunity. Breast-feeding is also vital for mother–baby bonding. What we do believe is that the womb and breast milk should not be contaminated by synthetic toxic chemicals in the first place, and so we encourage minimizing your exposure to them.

- **Intravenous**—A stay in the hospital can expose an individual to toxic chemicals such as phthalates (see Chapter 3), which can leach out of soft-plastic blood bags and medical tubing into the liquids (e.g., water, drugs, or blood) they contain and then into the patient.

How Do We Know What Our Toxic Body Burden Is?

The short answer is that we don't, unless we have ourselves *biomonitored*, and even then only a limited picture will emerge. Biomonitoring is a process whereby samples of blood, adipose (fatty) tissue, breast milk, urine, etc., are analyzed to assess whether certain substances are present and in what concentrations. It is virtually impossible for these tests to be exhaustive, because the number of chemicals that could be looked at is enormous and the process is expensive. Typically, a list of target chemicals is defined at the start of the biomonitoring, and the subjects are tested for levels of only those chemicals. These lists can be long, and they provide fascinating insights into the spectrum of contamination.

Knowing the extent of your personal body burden may encourage you to take steps to actively minimize your exposure to known and suspected toxic chemicals. However, where biomonitoring is most useful is in organized testing of the population as a whole to track "toxic trends" and to act as an early warning system for new toxic chemicals entering the environment and the food chain. Various NGOs (non-governmental organizations), notably the World Wildlife Fund, as well as governments such as Sweden's, have conducted "snapshot" biomonitoring programs that have provided a contamination overview—in some cases comparing regional, lifestyle, and generational factors. Though some studies are not large enough to be representative of the population at large, these studies have provided some interesting insights:

■ We are all contaminated, even in the womb—a location we idealistically associate with safety and the best possible environment for nurturing a developing child. A joint WWF UK/Greenpeace study of hazardous chemicals in umbilical cords tested over 30 newborn babies for 35 synthetic chemicals. The results revealed that between 5 and 14 of these chemicals were in their bodies already. Most of the chemicals detected are found in normal everyday products in the home (see Chapter 6).

In terms of our toxic body burdens, living in rural areas does not appear to be significantly better than living in cities. There is a prevailing assumption that rural living is more healthful and clean. Unfortunately, in terms of contamination with man-made toxic chemicals, this does not appear to be the case. What you eat (see below) and what chemicals you are exposed to in your indoor environments—your home, car, and workplace—may be more important factors than where you live.

The overwhelming majority of people tested by the WWF biomonitoring program had in their blood toxic chemicals found in everyday household products. It is impossible to say exactly how the chemicals entered their bodies. However, if people are living in intimate contact with these products, and the chemicals are able to leach out into the domestic environment, then this is probably a key exposure route.

PCBs, which are found at elevated levels in oily fish, are found at higher concentrations in the blood of people who eat more oily fish than in the blood of others tested in the same sample.

The WWF cross-generational biomonitoring survey of 2004 tested and compared toxic body burdens of three generations of the same families. The results showed that children were sometimes contaminated with higher concentrations than their parents and grandparents, despite the fact that children have had less time than older generations to accrue a body burden. While the older generations tended to have more of the "older" chemicals in their blood (DDT, PCBs, etc.), the children showed elevated levels of more "modern" toxic chemicals like brominated flame retardants (BFRs, used extensively in soft furnishings, electrical equipment, and textiles) and perfluorinates (common in non-stick pans, water-resistant clothing, and footwear).

Despite our extensive knowledge of how lifestyle factors affect our health and well-being, there is little we know with certainty about the dangers posed by commonly used toxic chemicals. However, there is sufficient evidence to warrant extreme caution. Until we know for certain what their health effects are, products that contain toxic chemicals need to be taken off the market or their toxic ingredients be replaced with safer alternatives. Meanwhile, the fact that these chemicals are not commonly labeled as hazardous, and often not labeled at all, means that we need to be as aware as possible in order to minimize our exposure.

CHAPTER 2

Sensitive Subjects

Many variables influence the effect of toxic chemicals on human health and well-being. A key factor is that we are all more sensitive to certain substances at some stages of life than at others. For example, a developing fetus is the most sensitive to, most vulnerable to, and least able to protect itself from harmful chemicals. Endocrine-disrupting chemicals (EDCs), commonly termed hormone disruptors, are particularly worrisome. A central problem is that established "safe" levels of exposure are primarily based on the effects of toxic chemicals on healthy, fully grown adult males. These exposure levels are then scaled down to account for effects on women, children, and infants. Also, many of these assessments are based on workplace and occupational exposures and do not really address personal or family exposure via the home environment. The shortcomings of this approach are the subject of much current research, especially with regard to chemicals that affect hormones, because their effects vary so widely depending on the metabolic process involved, as well as the sex and life stage of the subject.

Some individuals are far more sensitive than others to the effects of certain toxic chemicals. One person may develop an allergic reaction or a migraine after exposure to a particular product, such as a perfume, while another may experience no symptoms at all. In extreme cases, a small minority of people develop a condition known as *multiple chemical sensitivity (MCS)*, in which a wide range of allergies and intolerances occurs with low-level chemical exposure. This condition can be extremely debilitating, because it is nearly impossible to avoid MCS-causing chemicals and still live a normal life.

This chapter covers, first the critical issues of fetal sensitivity and the special vulnerabilities of infants and children and, second, the issue of why some people are more sensitive than others. It underlines, once more, why the only sensible approach is to use caution and minimize your exposure to toxic chemicals.

A Question of Dose

Back in the sixteenth century, a controversial Swiss physician, Paracelsus, coined the phrase "the dose makes the poison"—the idea being that the higher the dose of any particular chemical, the greater its toxic effect on living organisms. His ancient words still inform much of today's approach to toxicological assessment. However, recent research into endocrine-disrupting chemicals has shown that this is not always the case. A far more accurate assessment is to say that it is the dose plus the *timing* of the exposure that makes the poison.

Furthermore, scientists have discovered that, in some instances, extremely low doses of certain compounds can induce stronger toxic responses than higher doses—even when the test organisms are at the same life stage. In some of these cases, higher doses have no effect at all because, beyond a certain exposure level, there may be negative feedback, essentially cutting off any response. This is known as the "low dose" phenomenon (i.e., low doses are more dangerous than higher ones). A similar phenomenon is an "Inverted U" reaction, in which the toxic effect increases with dose up to a point and then falls off, hence the shape on a graph with dose measured along the bottom and response up the side (see table, page 26).

In some instances, extremely low doses of certain compounds can induce stronger toxic responses than higher doses.

This fundamental paradigm shift in our understanding of the action of toxic chemicals applies especially to those that affect the hormonal system and throws into doubt much conventional wisdom about "safe" levels of known endocrine disruptors. This new perspective is particularly critical to our understanding of the most vulnerable periods, such as embryonic and fetal development.

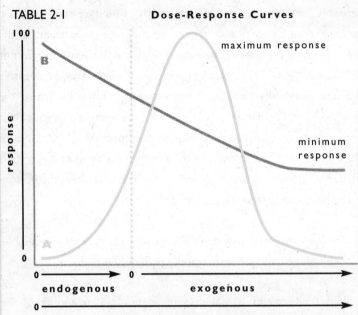

TABLE 2-1   **Dose-Response Curves**

The body's response to a chemical does not always increase with the dose. With some chemicals, the response drops as the dose increases because after a certain level of exposure there may be negative feedback (A), essentially cutting off any response. Or the response reaches a maximum, then falls off (B).

A Question of Balance

As touched on in Chapter 1, the endocrine system is one of the three major systems of the body and operates in intimate relation to the immune and nervous systems. The three must work in perfect harmony in order for us to be healthy and feel well. The hormones produced by the endocrine glands are powerful biological messengers, responsible for orchestrating development and behavior from the earliest time of cell differentiation in utero through old age. Their action is mostly taken for granted and goes largely unnoticed until the hormonal ravages of puberty, experienced to a greater or lesser extent by us all. These are a clear testament to the power of our hormones. The power of hormonal effects also becomes apparent when the endocrine system is undermined by external factors, such as chemicals that have the ability to mimic or disrupt naturally occurring hormones.

Endocrine-Blocking Chemicals

The endocrine system is a complex, finely tuned, and subtle messaging system on a molecular level, and its disruption can have far-reaching consequences on both physical and mental health. A number of synthetic chemicals are known to have the capacity to interfere with the normal function of the body's natural chemicals—the hormones—by blocking, imitating, or opposing their action.

Some of the most studied *endocrine-disrupting chemicals (EDCs)* to date have been high-production, high-volume, man-made chemicals such as bisphenol A and phthalates (see Chapter 3 for details). In some cases, these have been shown to have a feminizing effect, either by mimicking the female hormone (estrogenic effect) or stopping the action of the male hormones (anti-androgenic effect), and they are implicated in a range of conditions from arrested sexual development in males to accelerated sexual development in females. Research indicates that effects include lower sperm counts and rising rates of hormone-related diseases such as breast and testicular cancer. Other synthetic chemicals that are beginning to receive more attention are those suspected to disrupt thyroid and pancreatic function, such as BFRs and perfluorinates. EDCs are also being linked to rising rates of diabetes and other metabolically linked disorders.

> The endocrine system is a finely tuned messaging system and its disruption can have far-reaching consequences on both physical and mental health.

Early Development

Generally, the incidence of non-infectious diseases in children in the developed world is rising: conditions such as asthma, allergies, diabetes, and various autoimmune disorders. In some populations, there are also rising rates of reproductive system defects and anomalies such as lower sperm counts and earlier onset of puberty. Since immune response and primary sexual development are determined during prenatal and early postnatal development, much research has focused on this sensitive stage. Endocrine-disrupting chemicals and the "low dose" phenomenon have special ramifications for the fetus, infants, and young children—and, therefore, for chemical regulation. Governments have a responsibility to protect our young from toxic chemical interference right from the moment of conception.

Questions of Scale and Timing

In assessing the toxic effects of chemicals, infants and children cannot be treated as simply scaled-down versions of adults. Infants and children are very different from adults, both physiologically and behaviorally:

▪ Infants and children eat more food per pound of body weight, and therefore may take on a greater volume of toxic chemicals relative to their body weight.

Food stays in the baby's/child's digestive tract for longer, allowing more time to absorb toxic chemicals ingested in food. For example, a young child will absorb 50% of ingested lead, compared to 10% for adults.

A high percentage of the diet of infants and young children is cow or breast milk, which leads to a higher relative fat intake and higher proportions of lipid-soluble chemicals such as PBTs, as detailed in Chapter 3.

The blood-brain barrier, which limits the ability of most chemicals to pass into the brain's lipid content, is in gradual development during early childhood. So throughout this time, there is a greater risk of exposure to neurotoxic chemicals.

Infants and children breathe more rapidly, so are proportionally exposed to more air pollutants.

They have significantly different ratios of body fat to total body weight and water content to total body weight compared to adults, and a higher ratio of skin surface to body weight. Also, their skin is more permeable, so they are prone to higher dermal absorption.

Because of higher dermal absorption in infants and children, it is worth considering time spent in the bath, since water contains a variety of contaminants, in addition to whatever bathing products are added to the water.

Infants and children live differently, spending most of their time close to or on the ground, increasing their exposure to the various chemicals found in the house, in dust, carpets, and flooring, and outside on the lawn.

They constantly put things in their mouths.

They generally absorb chemicals more easily, process them more slowly, and eliminate them less efficiently.

A lot of children's clothes, including school uniforms and pajamas, are treated with perfluorinates (to make them wrinkle-resistant and/or water- and stain-resistant), brominated flame retardants (to protect them from fire risk), phthalates (often in those shiny plastic cartoon transfers on T-shirts and pajamas), and organotins (such as TBT, often impregnated into kids' socks as a fungicide). These chemicals are rarely identified on any labeling attached to the clothes. Taken together, they represent a potent chemical cocktail for the child (see full descriptions of these chemicals in Chapter 3).

Protective mechanisms at work in adults, such as DNA repair and the blood-brain barrier, are not fully functional in newborns or young children, and yet they are exposed to the same levels, sometimes higher, of toxic chemicals.

For older children approaching puberty, a time of raging hormones, mood swings, confusing feelings, acne, and fundamental physical and psychological change, the last thing they need is more chaos. However, an increasing amount of research shows that adolescence is often arriving prematurely, kicking off autoimmune disorders and diabetes, and exacerbating allergies and other problems.

Exquisite Fetal Sensitivity

The timing of exposure to endocrine-disrupting chemicals is critical to the developing fetus and young children, because the body's systems are most sensitive when they are under construction. During the early stages of development, important events are occurring all the time, providing many small windows of opportunity when the developing organism can be extremely sensitive to hormone-disrupting chemicals, such as during the formation of the testes (see below). This is known as *exquisite sensitivity* because of the almost unimaginably small amount of hormone that a fetus can react to. It has been shown to be as tiny as one part per trillion (a million times as low as one part per million). Any toxic chemical that can mimic hormones needs to be considered in the same light and treated as potentially toxic in infinitesimally small quantities.

A fetus may be sensitive to concentrations of hormone as low as one part per trillion.

DES: A Cautionary Tale

An example of the power of some EDCs is shown by diethylstilbestrol (DES), a synthetic estrogen prescribed to pregnant women in the U.S. between the late 1940s and the early 1970s. It led to many serious reproductive abnormalities in both male and female offspring, many of which did not become apparent until the children themselves reached puberty and beyond. Subsequent experiments on rats demonstrated how DES exposure at particular stages of fetal development led to reproductive system damage similar to that exhibited by the human victims. DES was a pharmaceutical product that superseded bisphenol A as the synthetic estrogen of choice until its devastating consequences became apparent many years later.

From Mother to Baby

Meanwhile, bisphenol A (see Chapter 3 for details) has made its way into a wide range of commonly used consumer products. Since the effects of many of these EDCs may be additive, exposure to several at low levels may have an effect similar to that of exposure to one chemical at a higher level. It's a disturbing fact of contemporary life that

KNOWN HEALTH EFFECTS ON DES
DAUGHTERS AND SONS

FEMALE OFFSPRING

- Clear cell adenocarcinoma (CCA). A rare type of vaginal and cervical cancer. Approximately one in 1,000 (0.1 %) DES Daughters will be diagnosed with CCA. The risk is virtually non-existent among premenopausal women not exposed to DES.

- Reproductive tract structural differences. Including T-shaped uterus, hooded cervix, cervical cockscomb, and pseudopolyp.

- Pregnancy complications. Ectopic (tubal) pregnancy and pre-term (early) delivery.

- Infertility. Difficulty becoming pregnant.

MALE OFFSPRING

- Noncancerous epididymal cysts. The most consistent research finding for DES Sons indicates that they have an increased risk for noncancerous epididymal cysts, which are growths on the testicles. In one study, 21% of DES Sons had noncancerous epididymal cysts, compared with 5% of unexposed men.

- Other genital abnormalities. A few studies have reported that DES Sons experience a greater likelihood of being born with undescended testicles (cryptorchidism), a misplaced opening of the penis (hypospadias), or a smaller than normal penis (microphallus). Because findings have been inconsistent, researchers cannot say with certainty that DES causes these types of genital abnormalities in DES-exposed men.

Source: Centers for Disease Control and Prevention, January 2007

regardless of lifestyle or location, an expectant mother will inevitably pass on a significant part of her toxic body burden to her offspring, both via the placenta and through breast milk. The placenta, essentially a barrier designed to protect the fetus, is robbed of this function when it comes to toxic chemicals of low molecular weight that dissolve readily in fat. And while breast milk is still considered best, it's sadly not as good as it used to be because of its accumulation of chemicals.

An expectant mother will inevitably pass on a significant part of her toxic body burden to her offspring, both via the placenta and through breast milk.

Very low levels of chemical interference can be catastrophic at very sensitive developmental stages.

Once across the placenta, the hazardous chemicals can mix into the amniotic fluid, which is constantly sipped and swallowed by the fetus. Then it can be absorbed by the digestive tract or skin, thereby leaving the maternal circulation and entering the fetal circulation.

The developing fetus lacks subcutaneous fat reserves, which can act as a buffer to lipid-soluble chemicals in older children and adults. Fat-soluble chemicals are more likely to end up being stored in fetal tissues that have high fat content, such as the brain.

The cells that produce sperm and eggs (germ cells) start to develop in the fetus and, in the case of males, mature during puberty. Chemicals can damage the germ cells, which may harm an adult's fertility and cause congenital defects in them or their offspring. More and more research is indicating that the male system is particularly vulnerable to chemical interference in utero.

The embryonic period, weeks 3–7 following conception, is a period of rapid development and exquisite sensitivity to chemicals, due to the early formation of organs and major systems.

Premature infants are particularly at risk of increased early exposure to phthalates because of the PVC tubing and other medical devices they get hooked up to in intensive care.

Sudden postnatal weight loss is not recommended, since this will mobilize the mother's fat reserves and release toxic substances into her blood and breast milk. Slow, gradual weight loss is recommended instead.

Male Reproductive Problems

Researchers have given the name *testicular dysgenesis syndrome (TDS)* to a collection of male reproductive disorders that are thought to have a common origin.

The TDS hypothesis is used to describe disorders that affect many males and are either apparent at birth or show up in adulthood. They are thought to be interconnected and linked to abnormal events in utero. The disorders evident at birth include failure of testicular descent into the scrotum (cryptorchidism) and incidences where the urethral opening is wrongly located (hypospadias). In many cases, both of these disorders require surgical correction. In adulthood, low sperm count, infertility, and testicular germ-cell cancer are becoming increasingly common in young men. It is generally thought that abnormal testicular cell development plus interference with the action of steroid sex hormones (androgens and estrogens) are probably involved, and that genetic, lifestyle, or environmental factors may help trigger the syndrome. The syndrome is the cause of much concern and has been discussed extensively in medical and scientific journals, including *Environmental Health Perspectives, Reproductive Toxicology,* and *The Lancet.*

The development of the testes occurs almost entirely during early development in utero where Sertoli cells, the cells responsible for producing sperm in later life, begin to differentiate. Exposure to estrogen concentrations at this time has been shown to reduce the number of Sertoli cells produced, possibly accounting for lower sperm counts in adults. There is also evidence to suggest that abnormal germ cells, formed in early development, are responsible for most testicular cancers in later life.

Several studies have documented that men with undescended testes and/or hypospadias are significantly overrepresented among patients with testicular cancer.

There is evidence that men who later develop testicular cancer have a lower proportion of male children (offspring sex ratio) than other men.

Although the endocrine-disrupter hypothesis is considered both relevant and plausible at the time of writing, relatively few chemicals have been closely examined for their potential effects on hormonal activity.

The seriousness of the problem is highlighted by recent health statistics from Denmark where trends in reproductive diseases, including testicular cancer, are showing a disturbing increase. Almost 1% of (mostly young) Danish men are treated for testicular cancer, an amazing 5.6% of schoolboys have undescended testes, and almost 1%

have penile abnormalities when they are born. Furthermore, over 40% of young adult men have subnormal sperm counts (Skakkebaek and Sharpe.[3]

Multiple Chemical Sensitivity (MCS)— Hypersensitive or Overly Sensitive?

A sensitive subject in itself, MCS is dismissed by a lot of people as a catch-all excuse for time wasters and hypochondriacs, and people who claim to suffer from it are often stigmatized. In general, the medical profession has been reluctant to legitimize MCS as an illness because there are so many factors that could contribute to the symptoms associated with it.

MCS SYMPTOMS

The symptoms of MCS are highly variable and include the following:

burning, stinging eyes	headache/migraine
runny nose (rhinitis)	vertigo/dizziness
sore throat, cough	poor memory & concentration
sinus problems	
wheezing, breathlessness	skin rashes and/or itching skin
nausea	light & noise sensitivity
extreme fatigue/lethargy	sleep disturbance
muscle & joint pain	digestive problems

What we do know for certain is that some people have much more extreme reactions than others to toxic chemicals in consumer goods. In rare cases, the reaction is so strong that the person cannot walk down the detergent aisle in a supermarket without his or her eyes streaming and skin starting to itch. Why this is the case is difficult to pin down, although there are plenty of theories. The standard industry canard that all these conditions are psychogenic or psychosomatic is increasingly being questioned by researchers in the field. It is worth noting that antibody-mediated conditions such as allergies and asthma were long considered to be psychosomatic until the real cause was identified. Along the same lines, research shows that certain enzyme deficiencies may explain some of the reactions grouped under the umbrella term MCS. This would explain why a chemical trigger can cause debilitating symptoms in one person while another will experience no discernible effects.

Antibody-mediated conditions such as allergies and asthma were long considered to be psychosomatic until the real cause was identified.

Allergy or Enzyme Deficiency?

It is important to recognize that people have biochemical and genetic differences that affect their level of tolerance to toxic chemicals and their ability to cleanse the body of certain chemicals. For example, lactose intolerance is often confused with an allergy to milk products, whereas it is actually a deficiency of an enzyme that breaks down lactose in the body. Similarly, several researchers into Gulf War Syndrome hypothesize that a certain percentage of the population lacks the enzyme to break down organophosphates, a chemical found in insecticides used by Gulf War soldiers as protection against insect-transmitted diseases. This could have serious ramifications for the producers of such chemicals.

Sensitization

Another critical aspect of chemical sensitivity is *sensitization,* the process by which the body becomes highly reactive to a particular substance after repeated exposure to that substance. In sensitization, an initial exposure causes the body to mount an exaggerated immune response. Since the immune system has its own form of memory, after sensitization has occurred, it will overreact every time the allergen or antigen is present. This can happen to allergens found in nature, such as pollen or certain foods (peanuts and strawberries are common examples). It can also happen from exposure to toxic chemicals. Occupational sensitivities are very common where chemical agents are used daily. For example, vehicle spray painters have very high rates of occupational asthma (90 times the national average). In Britain, occupational health statistics have shown that hairdressers, barbers, and beauticians have high rates of contact dermatitis (up to 16 times the average), and painters and decorators often have respiratory and skin conditions from prolonged exposure to the volatile organic compounds (VOCs) and solvents they use.

Not necessarily as debilitating, but far more common, are adverse reactions to synthetic fragrance—with even the briefest exposures capable of triggering headaches and other unpleasant symptoms like fatigue or difficulty in concentrating. The adage "one man's meat is another's poison" seems particularly relevant to perfume—one person will splash it all over and love it, whereas the next person will gag and run for the door for some fresh(er) air. In all of these cases, avoidance is the best policy. Unfortunately, this is increasingly difficult when so many common products contain such a wide range of chemicals. The task of identifying exactly which chemical triggered a reaction is made even more difficult by a lack of labeling. Again, self-education and awareness of which products cause adverse reactions are the keys to help you minimize exposure to those chemicals that simply don't agree with you.

CHAPTER 3

Common Toxic Chemicals: Ten to Watch

In this chapter, we will introduce you to ten of the most common toxic chemicals found in consumer products. This is not intended to cause sudden panic—we have to accept that toxic chemicals are frequently, if not always, present in our surroundings. Our goal, rather, is to inform consumers so that they can reduce their exposure to safer levels and can start to choose and demand safer, cleaner, greener options. Some toxic chemicals have been well studied and their toxic effects clearly documented. Of even greater concern are the many others that are added routinely to consumer products despite very little testing, making us all guinea pigs.

Since many of the following chemicals were developed to provide durability and convenience in consumer goods—making them waterproof, nonstick, or flame resistant, for example—and to act as preservatives, it is perhaps not a huge surprise that they have become such pervasive global contaminants. Some of the following compounds are PBTs (persistent, bioaccumulative, and toxic), some are endocrine disruptors, and some are so ubiquitous that our day-to-day exposure to them is pretty constant. Of course, among the tens of thousands of synthesized chemicals in widespread use, many more than these ten show worrisome profiles; we will make passing reference to some of the other less-studied compounds during the course of this book. It may well be that the vast majority of synthetic chemicals is "safe," but at the moment all we know for certain is that we don't know.

PCBs—An Example of How It Can Go Horribly Wrong

PCB stands for *polychlorinated biphenyl*. There are over two hundred variants of this compound. PCBs are classic PBTs (persistent, bioaccumulative, and toxic). First synthesized in the late 1800s, PCBs went into commercial production in the 1920s. They were swiftly adopted by the electrical industry when they proved to be supereffective insulators and coolants in electrical equipment due to their durability and nonflammable qualities. PCBs also found their way into the home in a whole host of consumer products where they acted as flame retardants and rubber preservatives, and were used as additives in paints, varnishes, printing inks, some pesticides, strip lights, and carbonless copy paper.

As early as the 1930s, there were reports of toxic effects in people working in PCB manufacturing plants, some of whom were developing an unsightly pustular skin condition called chloracne and complaining of other health problems. It wasn't until the mid-1960s that the wider consequences of PCBs first became apparent. Almost by chance, a Swedish scientist, Dr. Soren Jensen, who was investigating blood levels of another toxic chemical, DDT, discovered that not only were PCBs ubiquitous in manufactured products, but they were everywhere else too—rampant in the Swedish environment: in the soil, water, and animals. Further tests revealed them to be in Jensen himself, his wife, and his young children as well. On publication of his findings, the global scientific community began to investigate, and it became apparent that PCBs were disrupting food webs and contaminating environments all over the planet.

During this time it is unclear whether major producers and users of PCBs (companies such as Monsanto and General Electric) were aware of how toxic the product was that they were selling and discharging in huge quantities into the environment. It took over a decade, much litigation, and a huge body of research worldwide before Monsanto was finally prevented from manufacturing these hazardous, toxic chemicals (except for use in "totally enclosed" systems). Litigation continues to this day with respect to responsibility for various cleanup operations related to PCB contamination of the Hudson River, but the total fallout of PCB contamination will never be fully quantified.

There have been reports of young men rendered infertile due to their exposure; of related birth defects and developmental problems in exposed children; of legions of skin disorders; and of PCB workers dying of skin cancer. Dolphins have been found carrying over seventeen times the concentration of PCBs in their blubber sufficient to classify them as toxic waste. The Arctic has effectively become a dumping ground for PCBs and other persistent organic pollutants (POPs), the majority of which are *organochlorine* compounds released at lower latitudes by industries in developed regions like the United States and Europe. The compounds are swept into the Arctic by prevailing winds, diffusing quickly and easily into the atmosphere. Inuit women from Arctic regions, thousands of miles from any industrial source, have become so contaminated that many have to think twice about breast-feeding their babies because of the PCB concentration in their breast milk.

PCBs are so widely dispersed that they show up in the wombs of pregnant women and in whales in the deepest oceans.

Other studies on the health effects of exposure to PCBs indicated neurotoxicity (harmful to the nervous system, including the brain), reproductive and developmental toxicity, immune system suppression, liver damage, skin irritation, endocrine disruption, and probable carcinogenicity.

PCBs are classic "legacy chemicals," so called because they will continue contaminating the environment and living things for generations. They are so widely dispersed that they show up in the wombs of pregnant women and in whales in the deepest oceans, and yet there is no known way to get rid of them other than waiting hundreds of years for the gradual fading of their potent toxic effect. (A recent biomonitoring survey by WWF found that PCB levels in the blood were significantly lower than a decade ago, proving that strict regulation does work when properly enforced.)

The story of PCBs sounds like the fictional invention of a horror-story writer, but it's all too true. It demonstrates that no chemical should be put on the market prior to full testing to ensure its safety; that this should be the responsibility of the chemical manufacturer; and that strong regulations are needed to prevent companies from evading their responsibilities with legal loopholes. If a chemical is shown to be a PBT (persistent, bioaccumulative, and toxic), it should *never* go on the market to be used in consumer goods.

Even after the case of PCBs, classic PBTs, the lessons don't seem to have been learned. Chemicals with similar properties to the PCBs such as some brominated flame retardants (BFRs—see below) and perfluorinates (see page 48) are still in widespread use in everyday products. We need to learn lessons from the recent past, or we will all pay a terrible price.

1. Brominated Flame Retardants (BFRs)

Brominated flame retardants are synthetic chemicals that are added to many consumer goods, including furnishings, carpeting, bedding, children's clothing, and electrical goods, so that, in the event of a fire, they will burn more slowly. BFRs can be persistent, bioaccumulative, and toxic (PBT) and have endocrine-disrupting properties—particularly thyroid imbalances.[4] Negative health effects have been shown on the liver, the brain, and the nervous system when tested on animals.

When such chemicals are impregnated into products like mattresses and sofas, items we have close, long-lasting, and regular contact with, this is cause for alarm. Recently there has been a sharp rise in BFR levels in human breast milk. Where BFRs are shown to be persistent, bioaccumulative, and toxic, then humans, wildlife, and the environment should be protected from exposure and their use should be banned where exposure can occur. There is more and more evidence that the concentrations of some of these chemicals are on the increase in the environment, in wildlife, and in our bodies. In contrast to the flames they are designed to suppress, BFRs have spread like wildfire in the environment and are now a major global contaminant.

FIRE-RETARDANT FOREVER

As concentrations of BFRs build up in our bodies, are we becoming more flame-retardant in the process? This is not necessarily a joke. Plenty of anecdotal evidence from those involved in the crematorium side of the funeral business suggests that, for one reason or another, the modern corpse takes longer to burn and requires a hotter temperature than our ancestors did. While we're on the subject, those choosing the burial option may find themselves taking longer to decompose too, perhaps due to elevated levels of various chemical "preservatives" in our bodies.

It should be pointed out that there are legal requirements for certain consumer goods to be treated with flame retardants, although ironically it's the flammability of synthetic materials used in consumer goods that brought about these laws in the first place. (You may remember that when the first plastic TV and computer casings began to appear, they had a tendency to catch fire from the heat generated inside—around this time, manufacturers began to use cheap and available bromine to make flame retardants, and their use grew rapidly.)

Commonly, it is the polyurethane foam in soft furnishings, the plastic casings of small electrical goods like computers and televisions, and carpeting and floorings with synthetic fibers that contain the highest BFR content (up to 10% of the product's overall content in some cases). Many natural fibers, especially when tightly woven, and other natural materials do not require treatment with flame-retardants—or, if they do, it is to a much lesser degree. The presence of BFRs in consumer products has undoubtedly saved lives, and obviously we do not want people to burn in their beds, but the wholesale infusion of numerous common products with a proven global contaminant is an unwise solution to the risk of fire. Safer, less-toxic alternatives need to be developed for general use.

BFR Facts

The most common, most studied, and most worrisome brominated flame retardants are the PBDEs (polybrominated diphenylethers). There are three main variants: penta-BDE, octa-BDE, and deca-BDE— and over two hundred individual chemicals in the "family."

The European Union has banned penta-BDE and octa-BDE. The third common variant, deca-BDE, is still in use but is under constant scrutiny because there is the distinct possibility that it "de-brominates" into the more hazardous forms that are being phased out, and deca itself is suspected of posing health risks.

BFRs, particularly certain PBDEs, can rapidly build up in the environment and in living things, including humans. They are now embedded in the global food web and are showing up in ever-increasing concentrations in the blubber of whales from remote and deep Atlantic waters, and in the breast milk of women all over the world. Because of this, various governments, agencies, and organizations have urged adding PBDEs to the list of chemicals covered by the POPs Convention (see Chapter 6).

In some countries, the concentrations of PBDEs in human breast milk have been doubling every five years. Sweden took swift and early action, banning PBDEs in the '90s, and levels are now declining.

The European Union eco-label already prohibits brominated flame retardants, and Dell Computer has said it intends to apply for this labeling. Both NEC and Philips are working to replace brominated flame retardants in their products.

Health Risks

Chemically, PBDEs are very similar to PCBs, and both have structural similarities to thyroid hormone. PBDEs have effects on thyroid and hormone balance and are reported to have neurotoxic effects.[5]

Of special concern is exposure to PBDEs in utero, since these chemicals can be taken up during neonatal life, concentrate in the brain, and may have neurotoxic effects at critical stages of development.

Negative health effects have been shown on the liver, brain, and nervous system when tested on animals.

Where They're Found and How They Get Into Us

Common sources include sofas and other soft furnishings, carpets and rugs (especially those with synthetic fiber content), electrical goods (such as housings for computers, TVs, DVD players, mobile phones, MP3 players, PDAs), car interiors, public transportation interiors, offices, various textiles, and some clothing brands. They can even be found in some school uniforms and kids' pajamas.

There are two main exposure routes: first, through the food chain; second, via inhalation— as BFRs are widely found in the dust that collects on household floors and on objects such as computer keyboards. They are released from the objects that originally contained them and they contaminate both indoor and outdoor environments.

BFRs can also be passed to the fetus through the placenta and to babies via breast milk.

Healthful Alternatives

Buy from responsible manufacturers. Many companies, partly in anticipation of a possible ban on all PBDEs, are working to replace

BFRs with greener, cleaner alternatives. Major electronics companies including Dell, Ericsson, Philips, and NEC are all actively seeking and using solutions that are less toxic. Furniture-and-housewares retailer IKEA has phased out all BFRs from its products.

Minimize the products in your home that are treated with PBDEs; and when buying new goods, check for less-toxic or nontoxic alternatives. Choose tightly woven natural fabrics for your home (curtains, furniture covers, bed linens, and so on), and opt for wooden or plant-based floorings (like sisal or coir matting) instead of carpeting. Choose computers and other electrical goods with metal as opposed to plastic casings.

Keep house dust to a minimum and keep all rooms well ventilated.

To minimize exposure to BFRs, you could furnish your home with older, pre-BFR furniture such as antiques and actively pursue a preventative approach to fire risk (though this must be your free, calculated risk—furthermore, in some rental housing, furnishings may legally have to comply with fire regulations). To be safe, generally unplug electrical appliances when not in use (don't leave them on stand-by), install proper fire alarms, don't allow smoking in the house, and don't deep-fry at home—you know it's not good for you anyway!

2. Perfluorinates (PCFs): Convenient but Questionable

Perfluorinates such as perfluorooctane sulfonate (PFOS) and perfluorooctanoic acid (PFOA) from the group of chemicals that keep eggs from sticking to the frying pan, that keep the rain off our backs when we venture outdoors, that protect our carpets, shoes, and furniture from getting stained. These chemicals have strong water- and oil-repelling properties, are nearly impervious to heat, and are to be found in a number of well-known consumer brands of nonstick, non-stain, and water-resistant products. They are probably one of the most widespread toxic chemicals, and are found in us and other living things all over the globe, in levels that are increasingly a cause for concern. Because they do not degrade and are very persistent, they are sometimes referred to as "eternal compounds."

Exposure to perfluorinated chemicals such as PFOS and PFOA may cause birth defects, adversely affect the immune system, and disrupt thyroid function.[6] If exposure happens during pregnancy, other developmental problems may ensue. Our expanding knowledge about fluorochemicals in the environment again raises the question of how they could have spread so widely before being comprehensively studied by regulatory bodies. This is a classic case of industry not taking responsibility for its chemicals and not adequately testing them before putting them on the market.

If you have a canary in your kitchen, beware! Teflon toxicosis is a recognized and not uncommon cause of death among small pet birds. Even when used at "recommended" temperatures, nonstick cookware can give off toxic fumes that are potentially lethal to small birds. They die because the fumes cause their lungs to hemorrhage and fill with fluid, causing suffocation. At higher temperatures, nonstick fumes can sicken humans as well.

Perfluorinate Facts

▪ PFOS was voluntarily phased out of use in Scotchgard™ products by producer 3M in 2001 because of evidence of the chemical's toxicity. However, PFOA is still widely used in other consumer products.

▪ It has been shown that some fish can break down other less-toxic fluorinated chemicals into both PFOS and PFOA, which then persist and bioaccumulate in the environment.

The U.S. Environmental Protection Agency has recently come to an agreement with eight U.S. manufacturers to change their manufacturing processes so as to reduce emissions of PFOA by 95% by 2010 and eliminate trace amounts of the compound in consumer products by 2015.

There are serious concerns about the use of PFOS in fire-fighting foam, especially during big fires, where it inevitably contaminates the surrounding environment and water supply and may contaminate vast areas affecting many thousands of people.[7]

Health Risks

The U.S. Environmental Protection Agency considers both PFOS and PFOA to be carcinogenic, and occupational exposure to PFOS has been linked to increased occurrence of bladder cancer.

High levels of perfluorinates have been found in microwave popcorn packaging and have been shown to migrate into the oil in the popcorn during the cooking process. The same lining is commonly used in other fast-food packaging, but consumers have no easy way to know whether perfluorinates are being used.

Exposure to perfluorinated chemicals such as PFOS and PFOA may cause birth defects, adversely affect the immune system, and disrupt thyroid function. If exposure happens during pregnancy, other developmental problems may ensue.

If a nonstick frying pan is heated to over 662°F/350°C (some studies cite lower temperatures), it can cause a rare human disease called polymer fume fever. At high temperatures, the coating starts to break down into particulates and gases that can easily be inhaled, or ingested with the food cooked on the nonstick coating.

Where They're Found and How They Get Into Us

Perfluorinates are commonly found in waterproof outdoor clothing (such as hiking boots, synthetic "breatheable" fabrics, ski wear, etc.), wrinkle-resistant clothing (including school uniforms), carpets, upholstery, leather goods, floor waxes, nonstick cookware, occasionally inside ovens, and in aerosol cans used to spray stain protector onto shoes and leather goods. Perfluorinates are also widely used on the inside of fast-food containers, including those used for microwave popcorn, to stop the grease in the food from seeping through the wrapping.

The main exposure routes are thought to be ingestion via the contaminated food chain, through the inhalation of fumes, and via the general degradation of products containing them, polluting house dust and indoor air.

Concentrations of perfluorinates in some children are as high as in adults despite their having had far less time to be exposed to them. This may be partly because children play on carpets and floors more frequently, wear clothes impregnated with perfluorinated chemicals, and may be more sensitive to them.

Perfluorinates can also be passed to the fetus through the placenta and to infants via breast milk.

Healthful Alternatives

In the kitchen, choose stainless steel (the professional cook's choice), cast iron, ceramic titanium, or porcelain-enameled cast iron.

If you do cook with nonstick cookware, use at temperatures as low as possible. Keep the kitchen well-ventilated and, to be on the safe side, ensure that small birds, babies, and children are well out of the way!

Check the labels on your children's school uniforms for chemicals like Teflon, and choose natural alternatives wherever possible. If school regulations insist on certain suppliers, complain to the school administrators.

Avoid "no-iron," "wrinkle-free" types of clothing.

Avoid fast-food packaging, especially if it contains food with a high fat content—which is the vast majority of it.

If offered stain repellents when buying new furniture, say "no, thank you."

3. Phthalates—A Flexible Friend?

A strange-looking word, but a very common chemical. Phthalates (the "ph" is silent) are produced in high volumes in manufacturing, and are mainly used as *plasticizers* to make plastic products more flexible and less brittle. They are also used to give cosmetics that "super-smooth" feel. Not all phthalates are a health concern, but the ones that are should cause us great concern, as they are endocrine disruptors, implicated in a range of "feminizing" effects, and they are the classic leaching chemical since they do not bind strongly with the original product they are added to. The most common form, generally considered the most toxic, is DEHP. This is found in an extremely wide range of objects and places, including some children's toys, car interiors, PVC (polyvinyl chloride) flooring, blood bags, vinyl upholstery, shower curtains, plastic packaging, bags, all manner of molded plastic objects, and the ubiquitous credit or debit card.

Generally, the more soft and flexible a phthalate-containing plastic is, the higher the phthalate content—up to 40% of total volume. This is incredible, when you consider that a drum of industrial phthalate would carry a major health hazard warning and yet, up until comparatively recently, a child's teething ring could be one third phthalate.

While largely unregulated in the U.S. (other than a citywide ban in San Francisco), phthalates are now banned throughout Europe in toys and other products for children under three, and there are plans to ban more phthalate compounds in other children's toys and cosmetics. However, the effectiveness of this ban is questionable; it is suspected that many toys imported into Europe from places like the Far East are not checked and may contain the banned chemicals.

A secondary, but equally common, use of phthalates is as an additive in a vast range of cosmetics, personal-care products, pharmaceuticals, paints, printing inks, sealants, and adhesives—where their plasticizer properties perform functions such as preventing nail varnish from chipping and making moisturizers slide more easily over skin.

As flexible and prevalent as they are, phthalates are also very flexible contaminants, found universally in the environment, human body tissues, and fluids such as breast milk and semen. Despite not being particularly persistent in the environment, their commonplace usage means that they are a regular toxic guest in our bodies and that our bodily levels get replenished all the time—often from multiple sources. Some phthalates are known endocrine disruptors, and there is an increasing body of research implicating them in a range of health issues, perhaps most alarmingly with regard to male reproductive development in utero, general increases in male reproductive impairment, and the early onset of puberty and premature breast development in young girls (see Chapter 2).

Phthalate Facts

Phthalates have become one of the most abundant industrial pollutants in the world.

Products are not required to list their phthalate content on their label and often don't.

Although individual products may contain relatively low concentrations of phthalates, when you sit down and add up all the different intimate exposures you might have in one day (especially if you use a full lineup of personal grooming products), it is easy to see how levels can build up. This is especially true since phthalates leach easily from the products that contain them.

Although phthalates have a half-life of only around 12 hours, one study (Hoppin et al., 2002)[8] found that phthalate metabolites in the urine of women are generally quite constant, suggesting a constant daily exposure.

Health Risks

Some phthalates are known endocrine disruptors and have been linked to "feminizing" effects in men.

An increasing body of research implicates them in a range of health issues affecting male reproductive development in utero, general increases in male reproductive impairment, and the early onset of puberty and premature breast development in young girls.

One study in Puerto Rico suggests that high phthalate exposure during critical stages of development could be responsible for the high incidence of premature breast development in very young girls (8–24 months). One theory blamed the high volume of plastic-packaged food consumed there, combined with the constant high temperatures and high humidity.

Where They're Found and How They Get Into Us

Phthalates are commonly found in flexible plastics, such as molded plastic car dashboards, plastic food wrap, toothbrush handles, some toys including teethers and chew toys, car interiors, PVC (polyvinyl chloride) flooring, blood bags, vinyl upholstery, shower curtains, plastic packaging, plastic bags, all manner of molded plastic objects, and credit cards.

Many cosmetic products, including shampoos, hair sprays, nail polishes, and moisturizers, contain phthalates. When used as part of the fragrance (as a fixative), it does not need to be listed on the label.

As for how phthalates get into us, the short answer is "In every way possible":

- Ingestion, through biting and sucking objects with phthalate content and subsequent swallowing of the saliva (clearly this most commonly refers to infants and young children, but adult exceptions may also occur!)
- Ingestion, via food production and packaging
- Inhalation, from indoor air pollution and house dust
- Transdermally, from the legions of cosmetics and personal care products that contain phthalates
- Through an intravenous drip, if you receive medical treatment from blood bags or through flexible tubing
- From mother to child, through the placenta and from breast milk.

Healthful Alternatives

It's hard to avoid them, but manufacturers are increasingly advertising their plastics as being phthalate-free, especially those used in products for babies and young children.

Choose personal grooming products that are free of any petrochemicals or synthetic additives.

Choose natural flooring over vinyl (PVC) floor coverings.

Where there is an option, choose more rigid plastics over softer varieties.

Choose wooden or metal toys for your children.

4. Bisphenol A (BPA) or Polycarbonate

Although first synthesized as a synthetic estrogen (a man-made hormone), bisphenol A was quickly adopted by the chemical industry when they discovered they could transform it though the process of polymerization into polycarbonate, a plastic with many attractive properties such as low weight, high heat and electrical resistance, shatter resistance, and optical clarity. Endless uses beckoned, many of them within the food and drink-packaging industry. Possibly its only downside was that it was still effectively a synthetic estrogen and that the bonds locking it into the plastic could easily break, making it potentially quite a leaky chemical to use in intimate contact with food.

This glaring disadvantage does not seem to have slowed bisphenol A from rapidly becoming a nearly indispensable part of modern living. It's very big business, with almost three million tons being produced annually worldwide—and, like the phthalates, it's very hard to avoid. It's in thousands of products: from baby feeding bottles to mobile phones, DVDs to plastic lunch boxes, eyeglass lenses to the linings of baked bean cans—as well as in various floorings, composite building materials, paints, adhesives, and dental sealants. And of course, because of its leaky nature, it is in us too.

If bisphenol A had ever been introduced as a pharmaceutical product, it would have gone through multiple rounds of rigorous testing and had clear dosage levels attached to it. It didn't, because it was superseded by a more potent synthetic estrogen called DES (a drug that itself had disastrous consequences for many pregnant women and their children in the '50s, '60s, and early '70s—see Chapter 2). But as events turned out, we are all now getting varying and inadequately regulated doses of bisphenol A due to its widespread use in consumer products and the ability it has to leach from them into our food and drink, our environments, and our bodies. The levels we are exposed to and the impact on our health clearly depend on many lifestyle factors and our stage of life. Children are of great concern, particularly the developing fetus and newborn babies, given the use of bisphenol A in feeding bottles.

Bisphenol A Facts

BPA is in the epoxy-resin coating used inside some metal cans so that the food inside can be heated to temperatures high enough to kill any bacteria without the metal of the can contaminating the content. Consequently, many canned foods are now contaminated with bisphenol A instead.

Women tend to have higher concentrations of bisphenol A than men; this may be due to differences in exposure or metabolism between the sexes.

BPA is in seawater and has been found in many marine species that are eaten by humans.

BPA exposure is bad for snails, causing them in some cases to produce so many eggs that they burst.

Health Risks

Bisphenol A appears to have a complex and potentially insidious effect on the human endocrine system, with a possible ripple effect on the immune system. There are also indications that very low concentrations can produce negative health effects—especially when it comes to fetal sensitivity (exposure of the fetus in the womb through the placenta).

Although not without controversy, various strands of research have implicated BPA in breast cancer, male reproductive system defects, miscarriage, immune system defects, and polycystic ovarian disease. Recent research has also revealed a possible link to diabetes, insulin resistance, and obesity.[9]

Where It's Found and How It Gets Into Us

The vast majority of baby feeding bottles is made of BPA.

BPA is used to make plastic water bottles, baby feeding bottles, the coating on the inside of cans and other food packaging, plastic eating utensils, and plastic food containers, including the ones used in microwaves.

It's also found in a wide range of consumer products, including DVDs, mobile phones, electrical appliances, sports equipment, eyeglass lenses, some car parts, medical equipment, refrigerator shelves, dental sealants, flooring, paints, and adhesives. It's also present in certain pesticides and flame retardants, and is used as a stabilizer in synthetic rubber chemicals and PVC.

Ingestion is a major exposure route, because Bisphenol A is often in contact with food and drinks, particularly water and baby formula, and is known to leach from products that contain it. It is also released because polycarbonate plastics degrade over time.

BPA may also pass from mother to child through the placenta and breast milk.

Exposure also takes place by inhalation of house dust.

Healthful Alternatives

As with phthalates, pregnant women are especially advised to minimize their exposure. Use glass instead of plastic baby bottles. If polycarbonate bottles are used, discard them every three months or as soon as any scratches or other signs of wear occur.

Minimize intake of canned foods, especially those with a high fat content.

Use glass bottles instead of polycarbonate, especially for repeated use.

Do not microwave food in plastic containers.

For picnics and food on the move, try to use metal, glassware, and paper cups and plates rather than plastic.

Don't get white composite fillings at the dentist. Better still, pursue good dental hygiene to avoid fillings in the first place.

5. Formaldehyde

For many people, formaldehyde conjures up memories of sitting in a high-school science lab looking at a splayed-out frog on the biology teacher's dissection board, trying not to breathe in the horrible smell. So it will come as a surprise to find out that the same pungent chemical can be found extensively in home environments—in some carpet backing, curtains, flooring, and kitchen and bathroom cabinets—as well as in a range of products that have an even more intimate relation to our bodies such as lipstick, toothpaste, and soft drinks. It is commonly found in many brands of "diet" soda, where it is a breakdown product of artificial sweetener (see below).

Formaldehyde is a very volatile organic chemical (VOC). Even quite low-level exposure can affect the mucous membranes of the eyes, nose, and throat, causing burning and watering of the eyes, burning of the nose and throat, coughing, and difficulty in breathing. Higher and prolonged exposure can result in skin and lung allergies, and it has been strongly linked to asthma and various cancers.

Formaldehyde is produced worldwide on a large scale. In the form of urea-formaldehyde resin, it is extensively present in particleboard, interior grades of plywood and decorative paneling, and other pressed-wood products. Standard MDF, or medium-density fiberboard—that stalwart of the do-it-yourself home remodeler—contains the highest concentrations of any building material and emits the most formaldehyde into the air. (Low-emitting MDF and particleboard are available by special order in most areas. Use products that are certified as low-emitting by HUD or ANSI.)

Most plywood and composite materials used structurally in home building, such as exterior-grade plywood, waferboard, and OSB, are made with phenol-formaldehyde resin, which has negligible emissions. Large areas of particleboard, however, are often used as "underlayment" under carpeting or other floor coverings and can emit high levels of formaldehyde, as can decorative plywood paneling.

Formaldehyde is strongly associated with so-called "sick building syndrome" because of its extensive use in building products and its tendency to off-gas—which means it is significantly released as a gas, especially from new materials. Warm temperatures and high humidity increase the rate of off-gassing. Significant formaldehyde emissions can continue for as long as a year after installation and vary in concentration according to heat and humidity.

Embalmers use formaldehyde to preserve dead bodies and, strangely enough, it serves the same "preservative" function for the cosmetics industry in many shampoos, hand washes, bubble baths, and other personal grooming products of an aqueous nature. Exposure to formaldehyde in the general environment also comes from vehicle exhaust, smoke (tobacco, coal, and wood), dust, and vapors off-gassing from construction, insulation, and interior-decorating materials.

Formaldehyde Facts

Formaldehyde was a popular insulating foam for house walls in the 1970s, but was banned in the early '80s in the U.S. and Canada because of its toxicity to human health. (The ban was soon reversed in the U.S., but the product was rarely used again.)

Levels of formaldehyde in outdoor air are generally low, but higher levels can be found in the indoor air of homes.

Because of the large amount of particleboard and wood paneling in mobile homes, the Department of Housing and Urban Development (HUD) requires manufacturers to use low-emitting materials and to warn mobile home buyers about formaldehyde risks.

Health Risks

Formaldehyde contributes to "sick-building syndrome." Even low-level exposure can affect the mucous membranes of the eyes, nose, and throat, causing burning and watering of the eyes, burning of the nose and throat, coughing, and difficulty in breathing.

Higher and prolonged exposure can result in skin and lung allergies, and it has been strongly linked to asthma and various cancers.

The EPA and the International Agency for Research in Cancer consider formaldehyde a probable human carcinogen.

Aspartame (found in many table-top artificial sweeteners, diet drinks, diet food, chewing gum, etc.) breaks down into wood alcohol (methanol), which further breaks down in the body into formaldehyde, which, if regularly present, can cause gradual and eventually severe damage to the neurological and immune systems.

Formaldehyde is a known "sensitizer," meaning that some people can develop a heightened sensitivity to the chemical after repeated exposure.

Where It's Found and How It Gets Into Us

Common sources of exposure include particleboard, decorative wood paneling, MDF (medium-density fiberboard), and similar building materials; carpets; paints and varnishes; foods and cooking; tobacco smoke; and the use of formaldehyde as a disinfectant.

Formaldehyde mixes easily with water, but not with oil or grease, and is often used as a cheap preservative for aqueous personal grooming products like shampoos, hand washes, and even baby bubble bath.

Ingestion and inhalation are the most common exposure routes.

Healthful Alternatives

Avoid the use of particleboard as an "underlayment" under carpeting or other floor coverings. Avoid the use of interior wood paneling or any interior-rated plywood products. Wherever possible, use solid lumber or exterior-grade plywood.

Ideally choose alternatives to MDF or particleboard for kitchen cabinets, shelving, and furniture; but if you do use them, don't cut them at home without a mask and good ventilation. Seal all exposed surfaces with a low-VOC paint or sealer as soon as possible (see Chapter 4). If MDF is needed for a project, use the low-emitting type.

Try to install hardwood or other natural flooring instead of carpets or PVC. If carpeting is used, make sure it carries the CRI Green Label, which strictly limits formaldehyde and other emissions.

Use low-VOC paints, varnishes, and other wall and floor substances.

Choose toothpaste and other personal grooming products that do not contain formaldehyde as a preservative.

Don't allow smoking in the home or the car, since cigarette smoke contains significant amounts of formaldehyde (along with many other hazardous chemicals).

Drink plenty of water and fresh juices rather than "diet" drinks with aspartame.

6. Synthetic Musks

The human body apparently smells a little musky, especially when aroused, which is why the small but potent gland of an otherwise-innocuous miniature deer that lives high in the Himalayas became so plundered by mankind in our efforts to smell even "muskier" and be more attractive to other humans. The story goes that Henry VI was so addicted to the smell of natural musk that he died through over-indulging his habit of sniffing it.

International protection efforts and modern chemistry came to the rescue of the musk deer when it became a protected species; chemists managed to isolate its primary odorous element, muscone, in 1926. Synthetic musk was born. Real musk is still produced, but only about 700 pounds of it per year, and it costs roughly three times its weight in gold. In dramatic contrast, around 800 metric tons of synthetic musk are produced annually, and for a bewildering range of uses.

Synthetic musk is generally used as a fixative rather than a scent. As a fixative, its role is to make things like air fresheners, fabric conditioners, and body lotions—as well as actual perfumes—smell "better" for longer. The high molecular weight of synthetic musks, combined with their ability to blend easily with other aromatic ingredients, makes the olfactory potency of those ingredients more penetrating, more enduring, and deeper. So something doesn't necessarily smell "musky" if it has synthetic musk in it. The musk element is more likely to be there to amplify another smell, like violet, rose, or lavender—except in certain single-note perfumes where the bald intention is to try to create a sexy musky scent. Strangely enough, it is usually perfumes aimed at women that try to mimic the smell that derives from a sac that nestles next to the male musk deer's prostate gland.

On a molecular level, smell actually does touch your nerves; it is quite common for synthetically scented products to have acute adverse effects, triggering headaches, migraines, asthma, and allergies, and causing irritation to the eyes, nose, and throat. Strong scents are often described as "choking" and "eye-watering," and some people are clearly far more sensitive than others to these negative effects. Others can stand in a perfume counter all day squirting passersby while suffering no apparent ill effects. However, synthetic musks are both bioaccumulative and persistent in the environment. Some are known to be toxic, like Musk Ambretta and Musk Xylene, for example, and have already been discontinued.

Others previously considered only mildly toxic are being reevaluated in the light of some fascinating, if troubling, new research. There is a possibility that polycyclic musks, by far the most common, may act as "toxic enhancers" by debilitating cells' natural ability to defend against other toxic substances. If this is the case, considering that the plethora of products that contain synthetic musks often contain other hazardous chemicals like parabens, phthalates, and bisphenol A, then their toxic consequence could prove to be far more enduring and widespread than the smells they are there to prolong and intensify.

Musk Facts

The almost magical property of synthetic musk to enhance and prolong the smell of whatever it is added to explains its success across the spectrum of fragrance chemistry. Musk is to fragrance what MSG (monosodium glutamate) is to Chinese food.

There are three main groups of synthetic musks: nitro musks, polycyclic musks, and macrocyclic musks. Musk Xylene (a nitro musk) poses a particular problem, as it is a widespread contaminant of the environment. The polycyclic musks are thought to be less environmentally damaging than nitro musks, but they are toxic to reproduction. Macrocyclic musks are currently being investigated as possible substitutes for the other two musk groups.

AHTN and HHCB are the most common polycyclic musks.

Increasing levels of polycyclic musks have been seen in some samples of human breast milk.

Health Risks

A lot of people are allergic to perfumes. This can manifest in various ways, as skin reactions, headaches and migraines, general nausea, and irritation of the mucous membranes.

Synthetically scented products may have acute adverse effects, triggering headaches, migraines, and asthma, and causing irritation to the eyes, nose, and throat. Strong scents are often described as "choking" and "eye-watering." Some people are far more sensitive than others to these negative effects.

The polycyclic musks are persistent, bioaccumulative, and toxic to reproduction. They have been identified as possible carcinogens.

Recent research shows that both nitric and polycyclic musks may compromise the body's xenobiotic defense system, the basic defense mechanism that allows the body to defend against other toxic substances by pumping them out at a cellular level.

A number of nitro musks, a family of inexpensive synthetics used widely for decades, have been taken off the market because of their "photo-toxicity"—they become poisonous when exposed to sunlight.

Where They're Found and How They Get Into Us

Synthetic musks are almost as ubiquitous as phthalates and parabens, and are often found in the same products, especially those we use for personal grooming and skin care.

Wherever there is fragrance, there is usually synthetic musk. In addition to the obvious products such as perfumes, cosmetics, shampoos, conditioners, styling treatments, body washes, shaving foams, etc., they are also found in detergents, clothes conditioners, air fresheners, trash-can liners, children's toys, scented candles, toothpaste, candies, and almost every imaginable consumer product that manufacturers think can be made more appealing by adding fragrance, including chewing gum and ice cream.

Our exposure is typically through the skin and via inhalation of "fragranced air," although some is through ingestion of fragranced foodstuffs, toothpaste, and cosmetics such as lipstick, lip balm, and other products applied around the mouth area.

Healthful Alternatives

Use less perfume, or don't use it at all. It will more than likely repel as many people as it attracts. Also understand that in the vast majority of cases, it's utterly synthetic and laden with chemicals.

Purchase all-natural cosmetics and personal care products from reliable vendors such as Dr. Hauschka, Weleda, or Burt's Bees.

Use small quantities of essential oils if you need to add some fragrance to your products. A reliable natural-products company can provide them and can advise on appropriate quantities and combinations.

Avoid gimmicks like "fragranced" trash-can liners—just empty the bins regularly.

When shopping, be aware of the heavy fragrance added to hundreds of everyday consumer products, and always opt for fragrance-free versions.

 Ventilate the home rather than use so-called "air fresheners." Have an exhaust fan vented to the outdoors in each bathroom. Some people also strike a match to disperse bad smells.

 Avoid perfumed children's toys.

7. Parabens—Are You Being Well Preserved?

Parabens have been used as preservatives since the 1920s, to prevent the growth of bacteria in a wide range of consumer products, including a variety of foods and pharmaceuticals. Their most prevalent use, however, has been as a preservative in facial and body cosmetics, skin-care products, shampoos and conditioners, sunscreens, underarm products (antiperspirants and deodorants), colognes and perfumes, and soaps.

Parabens are cheap to produce and hard to avoid: the most widely used preservatives worldwide. Their rapid excretion from the body (in both human and animal testing) has led to a general assumption that their toxicity is of no real concern. However, more recent research has raised serious questions that point to the need for further testing.

This is based on over a dozen scientific studies indicating that several types of parabens can bind to estrogen receptors and cause estrogen-like responses. Other research showing that endocrine-disrupting chemicals can cause side effects at extremely low doses calls into question the safety of parabens, given their common presence in so many products that we use every day, often several times a day.

In addition, the recent discovery of parabens in breast tumors has led to speculation that they may be implicated in breast cancer (particularly since their action as an estrogen mimicker has been shown in research). The fact that most breast tumors occur in the part of the breast nearest to the armpit has led to further theories that parabens in underarm deodorants may be a culprit. This hypothesis has drawn currency from the fact that breast cancer is more common in the left breast, the idea being that because most people are right-handed, they apply more paraben-containing product to the left armpit. Although an interesting theory, it is unsubstantiated and much more research needs to be done. As a precautionary measure, however, it is probably worth avoiding paraben-containing deodorants and to avoid application of underarm products or other skin products immediately after shaving.

Paraben Facts

Parabens have long been used as preservatives to prevent bacterial growth in cosmetics, personal care products, pharmaceuticals, and some foods.

The four parabens in common use are: methyl-, ethyl-, propyl-, and butyl-parabens. Most products contain two or more of these chemicals as part of their preservative system.

Their rapid excretion from the body has led many people to assume that their toxicity is of no real concern. However, more recent research has raised serious questions about their safety.

Health Risks

Over a dozen scientific studies indicate that several types of parabens can bind to estrogen receptors and cause estrogen-like responses.

Parabens have been recently found in breast tumors, leading to speculation that the chemical may be implicated in breast cancer (particularly given their action as an estrogen mimicker).

Paraben allergic hypersensitivity is a form of allergic contact dermatitis that affects a minority of individuals. It appears to result from repeated contact with products containing relatively low levels of parabens, such as some cosmetics, grooming products, foods, and even children's gel-like play products.

Some cases have been reported of severe genital eczema occurring in men after they have used condoms impregnated with benzocaine and parabens.

Some Japanese research on methyl-paraben found that it did not metabolize in the strateum corneum, the outermost layer of the epidermis, and suggested that its presence accelerated skin aging.

Where They're Found and How They Get Into Us

Parabens are commonly found in cosmetics, shampoos, body creams, shaving creams, some deodorants, cosmetics, some children's gel-like play stuffs (like "slime"), condoms, pharmaceutical products, nail products, baby lotions, and bath products.

Parabens are sometimes used as preservatives in foods. On food labels, parabens will be listed as methyl p-hydroxybenzoate or propyl p-hydroxybenzoate. Parabens may be found in processed fruits and vegetables, fats, oils, seasonings, and such baked goods as cakes, pies, and other pastries.

Exposure through the skin is of much greater concern than ingestion, since the body's digestive system easily breaks down parabens.

Parabens have been found in breast milk, blood, and other body tissues, and they can cross the placenta and enter the developing fetus.

Although they are metabolized relatively quickly, like phthalates, our almost constant exposure to them means that they are generally in the body.

Healthful Alternatives

▦ Paraben-free options do exist and are generally found in health-food stores or in the "natural" product lines available in selected supermarkets and department stores. Always check the label first. Generally speaking, the four main parabens will appear in the list of contents if they are used.

▦ Simple emollients such as aqueous cream tend to work just as well as complex, highly fragranced, additive-laden "premium" beauty products. Also it's worth remembering that good diet, lots of water, and exercise will do more for your skin than any amount of face cream.

▦ A number of manufacturers are responding to consumer concerns over parabens and are developing preservatives made entirely from naturally occurring ingredients—for example, a Canadian product called Naturbak. However, it's difficult to find all-natural alternatives that will preserve things for the durations generally required. One solution is to have products with shorter shelf life, but this is unattractive to most mainstream companies.

▦ Choose all-natural product lines from reliable companies that go out of their way to avoid synthetic chemical ingredients and still manage to produce an effective range of goods.

▦ Generally streamline your personal care approach, use fewer products, and choose those with more natural ingredients.

8. Perchloroethylene or "Perc"

The phrase "being taken to the cleaners" refers to the bad business practices of the original "dry" cleaners, who would return garments smelling of gasoline and expect their customers to accept them. When you get your dry-cleaning back from today's chemical processes, you might be forgiven for thinking that nothing much has changed. Frankly, most dry-cleaning smells pretty bad, and comes back swathed in a layer of flimsy plastic that serves to preserve that acrid, unpleasant smell in your clothes, in your closet, and ultimately in you too. Ironically, it is usually our most delicate, natural-fiber clothing that tends to get the chemical cleaning—silk blouses, wool suits and coats, and so on.

Perchloroethylene, or "perc," is a chlorinated solvent and the most common dry-cleaning solvent in use. Originally developed as an industrial degreaser, it's been the staple of the dry-cleaning business since the 1930s. But, in light of recent evidence of the toxicity of perc, the dry-cleaning industry is increasingly seeking greener, cleaner alternatives. Perc is a very volatile organic compound, a hazardous air pollutant and groundwater contaminant, and causes effects in humans ranging from dizziness and nausea to liver and kidney problems—it is neurotoxic if inhaled in large quantities and is listed as a probable carcinogen by the International Agency for Research on Cancer (IARC).

Perc Facts

Perc is used by more than 80% of U.S. dry-cleaners.

The Occupational Safety and Health Administration (OSHA) strictly regulates U.S. workers' exposure to perc in dry-cleaning businesses.

In 2003, Southern California air quality officials voted to impose America's first ban on perc, which requires the phasing out of all perc dry-cleaning in Los Angeles by 2020.

Perc has been used as a general anesthetic agent because, at high concentrations, it produces loss of consciousness.

The majority of the dry-cleaning industry hangs on to perc as its solvent of choice, because it is such an effective product and because of the cost implications of changing. But at what cost to health and the environment?

Health Risks

Occupational exposure to perc has been implicated in higher incidences of cancer of the esophagus in several U.S. studies, and it is listed as a probable carcinogen by the International Agency for Research on Cancer.

Perc causes effects in humans ranging from dizziness and nausea to liver and kidney problems.

It is neurotoxic if inhaled in large quantities.

Where It's Found and How It Gets Into Us

The greatest exposure of consumers to perc occurs to people who live in buildings with dry-cleaning facilities, wear recently dry-cleaned clothes, or store chemically laden garments in their closets and drawers.

Perc is also found in some spot and stain removers, specialized aerosol cleaners, water repellents, suede protectors, and wood cleaners. Check the contents label.

The primary exposure route is via inhalation of fumes, but because of its persistence as an environmental pollutant, it is also in the water we drink and the food we eat.

Perc can also enter the body through skin contact, although this is less common.

Healthy Alternatives

▨ Don't buy "dry-clean only" clothing in the first place.

▨ Seek out less-toxic cleaning methods. In the U.S., a number of cleaners are switching to alternative methods such as the GreenEarth cleaning system, developed jointly by G. E. Silicones and Proctor & Gamble. The GreenEarth system uses silicone-based Siloxane D5. However, this is far from proven to be environmentally sound, since it is manufactured using chlorine and may be responsible for dioxin emissions. Research is currently being done on its potential toxic fallout.

▨ Liquid carbon dioxide is being adopted by some dry-cleaners as an alternative to perc. This technique, using special equipment made by COOL Clean Technologies, was rated as performing even better than conventional dry-cleaning by an independent consumer group.

▨ Use the new computerized "wet-cleaning" machines, which are able to control agitation and humidity levels to reduce the chance of shrinkage.

▨ If your clothes have been cleaned using a perc process, then remove the plastic and air out the clothes thoroughly before bringing them into the home or putting them away in your wardrobe.

9. Organotins

Organotins are a group of chemicals. Their structure consists of a tin atom attached to other atoms, including carbon. They are used as stabilizers or catalysts in PVC, silicones, polyesters, and polyurethane, as well as in glues and wood preservatives. One compound, tributyltin (TBT), was formerly widely used as an anti-fouling paint on boat hulls, to stop barnacles and other marine growths from attaching themselves to the metal hull, until it became clear that it was having a devastating effect on the marine life left in its trail. It was shown to have serious endocrine-disrupting effects on a variety of marine life. Its effect was perhaps most dramatically seen in the poor female dog whelk: when exposed to TBT, the whelks developed male genitalia and, in some cases, actually burst because they had no way to release the eggs they were producing.

It may therefore come as something of a surprise that the same chemical has been found in a wide and curious range of consumer products that includes baking paper (now withdrawn), plastic toys, and wading pools, as well as things in more intimate contact with the body such as insoles, socks, diapers, and the crotch padding of cycling shorts.

There are some concerns that the chemicals, which are persistent and bioaccumulative, can enter the body and attack the white blood cells on which the human immune system depends. Other concerns include the fact that TBT, a chemical compound that is known to disrupt sex hormones, has been found in disposable diapers. If a baby wears an average of five diapers a day, he or she could be in contact with up to 3.6 times the World Health Organization's estimated tolerable daily intake. Although its transdermal uptake has not been established, it is known that the chemical can be absorbed through the skin. The fear is that the chemical may be absorbed into the body and disrupt the child's sexual development, since very small levels have been shown to be disruptive to endocrine function. Although many manufacturers claim to have removed TBT from their diapers, it is worth checking, because it can be there almost accidentally as a by-product of plastic polymerization during the manufacturing of the polyurethane membrane used in some diapers.

Organotin Facts

The organotin TBT was, until recently, used in the anti-fouling paint on the majority of boat hulls worldwide. Because of its effects on marine life and the food chain, in 2003 TBT was banned by the International Maritime Organization (IMO) from marine use world-wide, and it will be completely phased out by 2008.

TBT is found in fish all over the world and in marine mammals including seals, dolphins, and whales, which are unable to expel it from their bodies.

Health Risks

TBT is a classic gender-bending chemical in nature, causing snails and female dog whelks to change sex.

The chemical may be absorbed into an infant's body from certain disposable diapers and interfere with the child's sexual development, since very small levels have been shown to disrupt endocrine functions.

Where They're Found and How They Get Into Us

Organotins are commonly found in disposable diapers, and are used in a similar way for sanitary protection in a variety of products. They are in inflatable beach toys like water wings and beach balls, in PVC flooring, in the plastic heat-transfer printing on team jerseys and other clothing, in sports shoes, and in household paints. They are also commonly used as fungicides in children's socks.

Organotins are found extensively in house dust; exposure can be through inhalation or transdermally.

Another major route is by ingesting contaminated seafood.

Because organotins exhibit PBT characteristics, they are also wide-spread environmental contaminants and are in our food and water.

Healthful Alternatives

Use washable diapers—they are better all around.

If you use disposables, select eco-friendly, biodegradable options.

If you do choose the bleached, additive-enhanced, mass-market options, then try to select a brand that states that it does NOT contain TBT (some carry the tag "certified TBT-free").

Reduce your use of PVC products, and don't buy children's beach toys made with TBT.

Don't buy clothing that promises "added fungicide" or that has similar labeling.

10. Triclosan

A product of our modern-day obsession with hygiene, triclosan is the chemical made by man to make as many things as possible anti-bacterial and anti-microbial. It gets added to hand soaps, toothpastes, and deodorants, and impregnates plastic chopping boards, trash bags, plastic kitchenware, and cleaning cloths. It's also closely related to dioxin, which happens to be one of the most potent synthetic animal carcinogens ever tested. Dioxin causes damage to development, repro-duction, and the immune and endocrine systems at infinitesimally low doses (in the low parts per trillion). Toxicological studies have not been able to establish a "threshold" dose below which dioxin does not cause biological impacts.

But that's dioxin. Triclosan manufacturers state that their product is safe, that it biodegrades and does not bioaccumulate. These claims are doubtful, however, given that triclosan has been found in human breast milk and has been detected in freshwater streams, in sewage effluent, and in fish from lakes affected by domestic sewage. It breaks down in sewage treatment plants to "methyl" triclosan, which is even more bioaccumulative; and, if you add sunlight to triclosan in sewage, it can convert to dioxin itself. Another bad characteristic of triclosan is that it produces highly toxic chloroform when combined with chlorine, as when a soap or detergent containing triclosan is mixed with chlorinated tap water.

On top of all that, in its original bug-killing function, triclosan probably contributes to the increased antibiotic resistance of bacteria in the environment, which has health implications for us all. Its undiscriminating, take-no-prisoners action on bacteria means that it also kills the "friendly" bacteria that occur naturally in our bodies and environment, and which aid our digestion, metabolism, and general ecosystem balance. Insufficient testing has been done on the wider effects of triclosan, but the singular fact of its chemical "lineage," along with its presence in breast milk and its questionable function (killing every bacteria and microbe around), means that it is best avoided wherever possible.

Triclosan Facts

The United States Environmental Protection Agency (EPA) has registered triclosan as a pesticide and gives it high scores both as a human health risk and as an environmental risk.

It has been estimated that triclosan's bioaccumulation factor is high enough to classify the chemical as "very bioaccumulative" according to criteria for chemicals of concern set out by the British government's Chemicals Stakeholder Forum.

One triclosan manufacturer proudly lauds it as the "aspirin" of anti-bacterial agents and boasts that it stays on the skin as a "secret protection" for hours after washing!

Health Risks

Anti-microbial formulas and disinfectants using triclosan can cause genetic mutations resulting in drug-resistant bacteria and mutant viruses, potentially producing new strains of harmful microbes for which the human immune system has no defense.

Under some conditions, it can convert to dioxin or combine with chlorine in tap water to produce chloroform.

Where It's Found and How It Gets Into Us

Triclosan is commonly found in anti-bacterial soaps, deodorants, toothpastes, mouthwashs, anti-acne medications, and foot-care products—as well as plastic cutting boards, plastic kitchen utensils, children's toys, socks, underwear, school uniforms, and bedclothes.

Ingestion takes place from mouthwashes and toothpastes, as well as from contaminated foodstuffs.

It can also be absorbed through the skin from soaps and skin-care products where it is used as a preservative, often alongside parabens.

Healthful Alternatives

There is really no reason to use products that contain triclosan in household environments. Just adopt a good and regular cleaning routine.

Be wary of clothing or bedding advertised as anti-bacterial; probably it is impregnated with triclosan.

Several retailers are already phasing out triclosan.

Sweden no longer sells products that unnecessarily use triclosan, and Norway is considering a complete ban.

Other Chemicals of Concern

Clearly, out of the thousands of chemicals used in common consumer goods, there are many more than ten chemicals that potentially pose a risk to human health. Most everyday cosmetics and personal grooming products contain a potent cocktail of parabens, phthalates, toluene (see below), and formaldehyde—plus a whole host of other chemicals. Since many of these chemicals have been inadequately tested, it is risky to start extrapolating from the scant research data and speculating about their effects. However, detailed below are some other toxic chemicals that are widely used even though big questions have been raised about their safety for humans, wildlife, and the environment.

ALKYLPHENOLS, ESPECIALLY NONYLPHENOL—These chemicals are used in great quantities on a global scale and have been used for over forty years as detergents, emulsifiers, and wetting and dispersing agents. Although the EPA has urged chemical makers in the U.S. to voluntarily phase out nonylphenol from detergents (and it was phased out of domestic detergents in Great Britain in 1976), these compounds are still extensively used in consumer products, shampoos, cosmetics, and spermicidal lubricants. They are not readily biodegradable and are known aquatic pollutants. The European Union wants to restrict nonylphenol as a "priority hazardous substance" on account of its persistence, bioaccumulation, aquatic toxicity, and endocrine-disrupting potential.

SODIUM LAURYL SULPHATE (SLS)—This very common chemical is found in shampoos, hair conditioners, toothpaste, body washes, and bubble baths. SLS started out as an industrial degreaser and garage-floor cleaner. When applied to human skin, it has the effect of stripping off the oil layer and then irritating and eroding the skin, leaving it rough and pitted. It can have terrible effects on the eyes, causing cataracts in adults, and is capable of inhibiting proper eye development in children. It can also cause mouth ulcers. But it makes products foam up better and seem super-soapy, and that's why SLS is added to common consumables. Best to check the label and select SLS-free products. If in doubt, keep well away from the eyes and mouth.

TOLUENE—This chemical has a variety of uses. In consumer products, it's often added as a solvent in paint, adhesives, and some detergents; it's regularly added to hair sprays, shoe polish, nail polish, perfumes, and cosmetics. When used by solvent abusers (glue sniffers), the excessive exposure can cause irreversible hearing loss and central nervous system and brain damage. In terms of day-to-day exposure, it is most likely to be absorbed transdermally by using personal care products that contain it or through inhalation of indoor air that is contaminated with it from nearby solvents. Chronic low-level exposure to toluene can cause irritation of the upper respiratory tract and eyes, sore throat, dizziness, and headache. Reproductive effects from exposure, including an increased incidence of miscarriages, have also been noted. However, due to many other variables, these studies are not yet conclusive.

METHYLISOTHIAZOLINONE (MIT) AND METHYLCHLOROISO-THIAZOLINONE—Regularly used as anti-microbial agents or biocides in personal care products such as shampoos and hand lotions, MIT and related compounds kill harmful bacteria that like to grow near moisture or water and are also often found in water-cooling systems. Recent laboratory-based research has revealed that even a ten-minute exposure at a high concentration proved lethal to nerve cells. This chemical is being used more and more extensively, yet there have been no neurotoxicity studies in humans to indicate what kind of effects it may have, despite clear indications that it could have neuro-developmental consequences.

MINERAL OIL—Like "baby oil," this is a petroleum by-product that coats the skin like plastic, clogging the pores. It can interfere with the skin's ability to eliminate toxins, thereby promoting acne and other disorders and slowing down skin function and cell development, resulting in premature aging. Any mineral-oil derivative can be contaminated with cancer-causing PAHs (polycyclic aromatic hydrocarbons—see below).

POLYCYCLIC AROMATIC HYDROCARBONS (PAHs)—Where there's smoke, there's usually some polycyclic aromatic hydrocarbons in the air. PAHs are ubiquitous environmental contaminants formed during the burning of organic substances such as wood, coal, oil, gas, rubbish, and tobacco. Initial concerns about PAHs focused on their carcinogenic properties, but more recent research has implicated them in endocrine disruption, toxicity to reproduction, and the ability to suppress immune function. There is also evidence that their effects increase synergistically when combined with other pollutants. In terms of consumer products, they are found in processed food and are produced by tobacco smoke, fireplaces, wood stoves, home barbecuing, and the charring and burning of food in conventional ovens. But even if you don't smoke, barbecue, burn your dinner, or have an open fire, the industrial activity in the outside world will ensure that PAHs are still present in your home.

CHAPTER 4

Indoor Pollution and How to Reduce It

Pollution is a word we tend to associate with grimy city roads, exhaust fumes, industrial plants billowing noxious smoke, and catastrophic events such as oil spills. We do not generally associate it with the cozy indoor environment we sleep in every night. Yet pollution levels inside the home can be as high as, and often much higher than, levels outside—even for inner-city dwellers. The types of pollutants found in the home can be very different from those we are exposed to outdoors, but they may still pose a significant health hazard. And then there are all the "on-body" pollutants to take into account—all those personal grooming products with their various blends of chemicals given direct access to our skin. Since we spend so much of our time inside—at home, in the car, or at work—it's important to know the sources of indoor pollution and how to reduce pollution levels in indoor environments.

Modern trends in home construction—tightly sealed windows and doors, heavy insulation, air and vapor barriers, and high-efficiency heating systems—all contribute to keeping indoor air inside. These are all good for keeping out the cold, but not so appealing when you consider the potent cocktail of volatile organic compounds (VOCs) and other chemicals that may be off-gassing from paints and other finishes, particleboard and MDF, carpeting, various plastics, the flame retardants in soft furnishings, electronic products and gizmos, phthalates in PVC flooring, and various other home products. Plus there will be sporadic surges of airborne chemicals after cooking with nonstick cookware, scouring the house with super-strength cleaners, or spraying air fresheners or stain repellents. Even the effect of high air temperatures on a hot summer day can make toxic chemicals more volatile than usual.

While there are clear energy-saving benefits to tightly sealed windows and high levels of home insulation, it is absolutely essential to have outdoor air flowing into the home to reduce the concentrations of any airborne contaminants. Having a house full of chemically laden fixtures, furnishings, and products in a near-airtight environment makes for a very unhealthful living situation.

The Importance of Ventilation

In areas with relatively clean outdoor air, a quick and easy way to reduce indoor pollution, in the short term, is to open a few windows to promote ventilation and air circulation. This time-tested approach to ventilation still has merit, particularly when indoor pollutant levels are temporarily raised by activities such as painting, cleaning with strong household chemicals, or certain crafts and hobbies. In areas where security is an issue, locks can be installed that allow the windows to remain open for ventilation but closed to intruders. However, in most parts of the U.S., windows are kept closed much of the year for energy savings (or in some case, allergy prevention). In these houses, mechanical ventilation is the best approach to ensuring a reliable supply of fresh air throughout the year. Ventilation systems are particularly important in newer homes, which are built significantly more airtight than homes built just a generation ago (see "Build Tight, Ventilate Right").

Clearly there are exceptions to wanting to bring the outside air into your home: for example, if you live next to a waste incinerator or a huge industrial plant, or in a basement apartment next to a busy road. In these situations you don't want to use outdoor air for ventilation purposes unless it can be effectively filtered before it enters the home. In some cases, air cleaners can be used effectively to filter air already being circulated inside the home. This is an option worth considering for people with strong allergies, asthma, or special sensitivities (see "What About Air Cleaners?").

BUILD TIGHT, VENTILATE RIGHT

Since the energy crisis in the 1970s, U.S. homes have been built increasingly tighter, due to changes in codes, materials, and standard practices. Even in the absence of special efforts to build airtight, simply using modern building materials, such as doors and windows with tight seals, plastic building wraps, sill seals, and foam sealants, adds up to a much tighter shell. Studies have consistently shown that many new homes are built so tight that they do not meet consensus national standards for fresh air (see below).

And even homes that are theoretically leaky enough to provide ventilation cannot be relied on to ventilate when and where you need it. Natural air leakage is greatest on windy days and very cold days, not necessarily when the most ventilation is needed. And there's no control over air distribution or the source of the "fresh" air, which may be a musty crawlspace. The only reliable way to guarantee adequate ventilation throughout the year is to build a tight house and to control the air flow with a mechanical ventilation system. The best systems are designed to pull air out of kitchens, bathrooms, laundries, and other sources of moisture and pollutants, and deliver fresh air to bedrooms and other living areas.

The simplest system, which can be effective for small homes, is a centrally located quiet bathroom exhaust fan operated by a timer to run intermittently throughout the day (with a manual override for bathroom use). Doors should be undercut to allow for air to circulate. More sophisticated systems use ductwork to exhaust air from kitchen, bathrooms, and laundries, and deliver air to bedrooms and main living areas. Some of these systems, called *heat recover ventilators*, use both exhaust and supply fans and reclaim some of the heat (or cooling) from the exhaust airstream.

One advantage of systems that use supply fans is that the air can be filtered before entering the home. This is a big advantage in areas

(continued)

(Build Tight, Ventilate Right continued)

where the outdoor air is polluted or filled with allergens such as pollen.

With ventilation systems that rely solely on exhaust fans, it is important to make sure that all the home's exhaust fans, when run at the same time, do not cause combustion devices to *backdraft*, that is, pull fumes back into the house from water heaters, boilers and furnaces, or fireplaces and wood stoves. Use a qualified contractor to install ventilation equipment and to test for any potential backdrafting problems.

VENTILATION STANDARD

The minimum ventilation rate recommended for single-family homes is 7.5 cfm per person (based on the number of bedrooms, plus one) plus a factor of .01 cfm for each square foot of household living space. For example, a 3-bedroom, 1,500 sq. ft. house should have (4 x 7.5) + (.01 x 1,500) or 45 cfm of continuous ventilation. This is based on ASHRAE Standard 62.2 (2003). This is recommended for all homes and is required under some state building and energy codes.

For a good comparison of different options for residential ventilation, see *Recommended Ventilation Strategies for Energy-Efficient Production Homes*, by Judy A. Roberson et al., Lawrence Berkeley Laboratory, 1998. This report can be found online at *http://enduse.lbl.gov/projects/ESVentilation*.

WHAT ABOUT AIR CLEANERS?

Want clean air? The logical answer, it may seem, is to buy an air cleaner. Like most mechanical devices, however, this can help in some cases but is no panacea. How effective a unit is depends on its size, type of filter, location, and how well it is maintained. In general, small tabletop units provide little help. Larger "console"-style units (air-conditioner size) may be effective in one or two rooms— potentially a good strategy for a person with strong allergies or sensitivities. Systems built into the home's main ductwork have a whole-house effect, but work only when the furnace/AC fan is running. These whole-house systems may reduce household *particulate* (small airborne particle) levels by up to a third, but may not have much effect on allergens like animal dander, visible dust, and pollen, which are heavy particles often found settled on surfaces. A vacuum equipped with a high-efficiency HEPA filter is the best way to remove these irritants from the home.

Also, remember that filters remove only particles from the air, not gases such as formaldehyde, VOCs, or combustion fumes. Some types of special media like activated charcoal may reduce certain odors or gases, but this is not a reliable strategy for providing clean air.

The main types of filter elements, with their pros and cons, are described below. Most of these filter types can be installed in the central heating/cooling system, or they may be available in standalone units serving one or two rooms. With all filter types, regular replacement or cleaning is required for the unit to do its job.

Flat filters. The typical "furnace filter" is inexpensive, but mainly removes large, visible dust particles. It has little effect on the smaller particles (particulates) that may be associated with health problems. They are inexpensive, but must be replaced frequently.

(continued)

(*What About Air Cleaners?* continued)

Pleated filters. Depending on their efficiency, these can remove 20% to 50% of particulates from the air passing through. Cost varies with efficiency. Look for a "dust spot efficiency" rating of at least 25%. Replacement is required every 3 to 12 months.

Electrostatic. These are typically plastic elements, permanently charged with static electricity. They are slightly more effective than a standard furnace filter, but must be cleaned frequently to maintain their effectiveness.

Electronic. These use a series of electrically charged metal plates or special filters to remove particles from the air. They are very effective against both large and small particles if the filter is cleaned regularly. These are a good choice for people with allergies. They are costly, but the filter is reusable.

HEPA filters. These high-efficiency filters catch the smallest particles, including spores, mites, and some viruses. Because of their high resistance to airflow, they typically require a separate fan and often include a pre-filter to prevent clogging. These are a good choice for people with allergies or chemical sensitivities. They are the most costly filters and typically last 1–3 years.

In all situations, ventilation or filtration can help improve indoor air quality, but they are intended only as backup strategies. The primary strategy to make your indoor environment as fresh and chemical-free as possible should always be to keep toxic chemicals out of the home in the first place. And if they must be used, try to restrict their use to contained areas with adequately powered exhaust fans.

Assessing Your Home

Whatever your situation, it's worth making a step-by-step assessment of the toxic potential of your indoor environments. Then draw up:

 a **short-term strategy** for products you can easily eliminate or replace with less-toxic alternatives;

 a **medium-term strategy** for reducing your exposure to the more volatile organic compounds and other toxic chemicals in your home; and

 a **long-term strategy** for when you can make bigger changes such as replacing flooring or furniture, or even moving to a new home.

If you've read this book up to this point, you'll have a pretty good idea of what chemicals are found where in consumer products and in the domestic environment. This chapter is a guide to the most common sources of indoor pollution and offers suggestions for alternative products.

Everyone's home environment is different, and it's a good idea to make an educated assessment of your health and the health of others in your household. If there's a high incidence of headaches, dizziness, and general fatigue, or if people simply report feeling better when they leave the home, indoor pollution may be a problem and steps should be taken to reduce it. Also, some individuals may feel worse after using certain cleaning products or spraying air freshener or perfumes. Often we attribute these adverse reactions to "some virus or other," or to other lifestyle factors such as working too hard or too many late nights, when it may well be pollution at home. Symptoms such as headaches; eye, nose, and throat irritation; allergies; and asthma are acute symptoms that are often more or less immediate reactions to contaminants. In addition, there are many chronic effects that can result from long-term consistent exposure. This may lead to respiratory disease, heart disease, immune disorders, reproductive defects, and cancer. People will react in a variety of ways to different toxic chemicals, babies and children being especially vulnerable.

House Dust

The presence in house dust of most of the toxic chemicals mentioned in this book is a good indicator of the indoor levels of contaminants. It also casts doubt on various manufacturers' claims that dangerous chemicals are safely bound into products and therefore do not present an exposure threat. In a major analysis of house dust performed by Greenpeace in 2003, it was found that all dust samples (from 100 homes in ten different regions across the UK) contained brominated flame retardants, phthalates, and organotins, in addition to a whole range of VOCs and other solvent and plastic additives.

A Greenpeace analysis of dust samples from 100 homes found that *all* contained toxic chemicals.

Dust in the home represents a significant direct exposure route for humans; it is a particular threat to children. The received wisdom that house dust is just an accumulation of dead skin cells and random dirt particles is no longer accurate; given its toxic content, care should be taken when disposing of it from dustpans or vacuum cleaners. As an indicator of the scale of contamination of our homes, dust is a lowly but important signifier. And while we may be motivated to vacuum and dust more diligently in light of these findings, in the long term we should insist that manufacturers use less-leaky and less-toxic chemicals in products destined for our home environments.

Carpeting and Your Health

Wall-to-wall carpeting has become by far and away the most popular residential floor covering in much of the U.S. While carpeting offers many advantages in comfort, convenience, and sound deadening, there are a number of reasons to consider other flooring options. Although it has been embraced as an easy, hassle-free floor covering, apart from harboring dust and dust mites, carpeting is often heavily treated with brominated flame retardants, stain resistors (perfluorinated chemicals), anti-microbial treatments (organotins), formaldehyde (usually in the glue backing), and various pesticides—all of which may off-gas or leach into the household air.

Furthermore, the carpet pile tends to attract and harbor airborne particles, including pollutants from VOCs, synthetic fragrances, paints, and cleaning products, plus all the pollutants brought in on shoes from outdoors, including toxic lawn chemicals. Aside from the common toxic chemicals detailed in this book, old carpets have also been found to contain high concentrations of heavy metals such as lead, cadmium, and mercury, polyaromatic hydrocarbons, and PCBs. Carpets also collect pet allergens, heavily implicated in childhood allergies and asthma, which are then spread from place to place on occupants' clothes. British researchers at the Manchester Asthma and Allergy Study Group reported in *The Lancet* that "environmental manipulation," including removing carpets from infants' bedrooms, reduced symptoms of asthma and allergies in high-risk babies. Because of these problems, Sweden does not allow wall-to-wall carpeting in schools, public buildings, or offices.

In the U.S., the first highly publicized case of "sick-building syndrome" occurred when new carpeting was installed at the U.S. EPA's headquarters in Washington, D.C., in 1988, leading to widespread health problems among workers there. Responding to consumer concerns and EPA pressure, the Carpet and Rug Institute launched a voluntary testing and labeling program in 1992, called the Green Label program, which now certifies carpets and adhesives that meet a low-emitting standard set by the industry. Their new Green Label Plus program meets the more stringent criteria of California's Collaborative for High Performance Schools (CHPS), a model design code for new healthful schools in the state.

If you do have wall-to-wall carpets throughout the home, it is important to keep your home well ventilated and the carpet well vacuumed (making sure not to overfill the bag or collection chamber!). It's important to make sure that your vacuum cleaner is up to the job. A central vacuum system that vents to the exterior is a good option. For occupants with allergies or special sensitivities, a HEPA-rated vacuum may be a good investment. Whatever type you use, if it's not well sealed, then it's liable to kick up the dust and redistribute it around the room and into the air. Carpeting can hold up to eight times its own weight in dirt, so clearly the deeper the pile, the more toxic it can be. Some newspapers have even dubbed carpets "the toxic sponge."

Carpeting can hold up to eight times its weight in dirt.

If you are considering installing carpeting, or even using area rugs, try to have them sufficiently aired out before being installed, and avoid gluing them down. The "stretch-in" method, using tack strips, is a better option. Choose a naturally flame-retardant product like tightly woven wool with a natural backing such as jute, or a hemp-and-cotton mix containing natural stain inhibitors such as lanolin from fleece. In the bigger environmental picture, carpets and rugs such as these are also biodegradable at the end of their service life. If you do choose a synthetic carpet, look for products (carpet, pads, and adhesives) certified as low-emitting by the "Green Label" or "Green Label Plus" program of the Carpet and Rug Institute (CRI).

PVC Flooring

If you have wall-to-wall carpets in most of your home, *and* vinyl (PVC) flooring everywhere else, you're living with one of the most toxic combinations underfoot. It is especially important to review these flooring choices if you have young children, because of their usual closeness to ground level and their susceptibility to asthma and allergies. Vinyl flooring contains phthalates, chlorinated paraffins, and possibly lead or tin compounds as stabilizers. The phthalates leach into house dust and into the air, and they transfer to the water used to clean the flooring. PVC has been associated with increased risk of asthma, based on a Nordic survey that linked exposure to plasticizers (chemicals used to soften PVC) to inflammation of the airways. Many countries already restrict the use of PVC in public buildings because of health and environmental risks. Linoleum, wood, rubber, and other alternatives are just as hard-wearing and as easy to maintain as carpet and PVC, and are much less likely to accumulate allergens. Furthermore, dioxin is created in the manufacture of PVC, and is created again if it's destroyed by incineration.

HEALTHFUL FLOORING OPTIONS

Wood. Choose species from sustainable forests. If you select wood laminates, insist on low- or zero-emitting boards. Choose low-VOC finishes.

Natural linoleum. Naturally anti-bacterial, antistatic, and resistant to fats and oils. Linoleum is long-lasting, low-maintenance, and made from renewable materials.

Bamboo. It's a very renewable resource, but check on preservatives; low-toxicity boric acid is best.

Natural rubber. Another good renewable resource, with good durability and sound absorption, although you should avoid rubber flooring with chlorinated content.

Rugs or carpet. If you want rugs or carpets, try to select those with vegetable fiber content, since they are not sprayed to protect against animal-borne diseases like anthrax (particularly from Eastern nations) or with other pesticides. Look for sisal, coir, or seagrass. Choose a tight weave for natural flame retardance, and seek out those with a natural backing.

Use a doormat at the front door and try not to wear shoes around the home.

Toxic Slouch and Slumber

The simple enjoyment of snuggling up in bed, or on the sofa, may be compromised if you realize how much toxic chemical content can be nestling there in the fibers just inches from your nose. Bedding, soft furnishings, mattresses, cushions, and pillows can be heavily treated with a range of chemicals, from the ubiquitous flame retardants through stain guards, organotins, and even synthetic musks. Wrinkle-free bedding may contain formaldehyde, the ticking on your mattress may contain PVC, and the whole surface might contain perfluorinates for water and stain resistance (especially children's mattresses).

Labeling of contents is often wholly inadequate, and the only way to ensure a chemical-free or -reduced product is to buy from a reliable vendor who guarantees that their products are non-toxic. Since we spend so much time in bed, often in intimate skin contact with bedding materials, it is worth investing in combinations of natural products, organic cottons, latex, and natural wool. Natural fibers are more tightly woven, and more naturally flame retardant, than synthetics. These natural bedding materials give off far fewer emissions than those made with polyurethane foams and vinyl coverings. Polyester sheets and nightwear, apart from the alarming habit of generating static electricity sparks as you slide into them, are also not very healthful sleeping partners.

SAFE SLEEP TIPS

- Choose organic cotton mattresses and bedding that allow you and your skin to breathe easily wherever possible.

- Buy from manufacturers that have found alternatives to brominated flame retardants.

- Avoid gimmicks such as "fragranced" pillows or other bedding.

- Don't have bedding dry-cleaned, but if you absolutely have to and can't find a perc-free service, then be sure to air it out well before using it.

- Keep your bedroom well ventilated and as free as possible of consumer products such as computers, televisions, fragranced candles, carpeting, and perfumed products.

- Be especially vigilant about the content of your baby's cot and mattress. This is the last place to compromise, since an infant's airways are smaller and more vulnerable to allergens and toxic chemicals.

- If you are unsure about the content of new mattresses, let them off-gas in a well-ventilated room before sleeping on them.

High-Tech and Toxic

Modern technology has given us a vast array of electronic devices to entertain ourselves with and to use to communicate with others while at home. TVs, DVD players, VCRs, PDSs, MP3 players, game consoles, stereo systems, plasma screens, laptop and desktop computers, home movie projectors, and cordless and cell phones are all commonplace domestic gadgets, often regardless of socio-economic background. Viewed from a health perspective, they are a mass of plastic casings, semi-conductors, and liberal quantities of chemicals, including the ubiquitous phthalates, formaldehyde, and brominated flame retardants.

These chemicals off-gas into the indoor air; the longer the products are turned on and the hotter they get, the more they off-gas—especially if the products are new. The chemicals also leach out of the products into house dust that settles on objects and on flooring and that inevitably circulates in the air as we move about, disturbing the dust. In the broader environmental context, the disposal of defunct or unwanted "e-waste" is a huge problem. Much of the content cannot be disposed of safely or recycled. Pressure needs to be put on manufacturers to develop safer, more sustainable, less-toxic alternatives, but meanwhile:

Try to purchase from manufacturers that are committed to researching and using greener, cleaner chemicals in their products (and do your own research, since the list is expanding all the time).

Choose metal or wood casings over plastic wherever possible.

Turn electrical goods off when not in use.

Don't let them overheat.

Make sure the rooms where they are used are well ventilated—particularly while electrical goods are still new.

Keep these products to a minimum. Resist the temptation to upgrade your phone/MP3 player/PDA every few months—newer products off-gas more than older ones, and it's environmentally irresponsible to frequently discard so many items.

Cleaners Not So Clean

Products sold as cleaners can be pretty dirty. Take the black scum that collects in your washing-machine soap and bleach receptacles, for example. There are multiple chemicals that go into the various high-power degreasers, drain decloggers, oven cleaners, floor cleaners, and conditioning fluids, and often there is a strong synthetic fragrance to cover up the noxious chemical smell that would otherwise prevail. Countless individuals are sensitive to cleaning products, breaking out in lumps and bumps or experiencing headaches, nausea, and irritated mucous membranes. The simple answer is to completely review the list of products you use to clean and freshen your home. Try to use fewer products, select "green" brands, and use more of your own muscle. Appreciate the fact that the greater the variety of products you regularly use, the more complex will be the chemical cocktail that you are exposing yourself and other household members to. Cleaning agents emit volatile organic compounds (VOCs), including formaldehyde. They also regularly contain phthalates, synthetic musks, and triclosan—chemicals that can pose a wide range of hazards to human health, including cancer.

What Might Be Lurking Under Your Sink?

OVEN CLEANERS contain powerful and corrosive alkaline agents, such as sodium hydroxide or potassium hydroxide. A single exposure can severely burn the skin and damage the eyes. Aerosols are worse, since a mist of the caustic chemicals can drift onto skin, eyes, and sensitive lung surfaces. Most oven cleaners do warn that they can burn skin and eyes and that fumes and vapors should be avoided. If you can't avoid using these products, do take their warnings seriously. Ensure proper ventilation, and wear a mask and rubber gloves.

WASHING POWDERS (especially the "biological" kind) are often based on a corrosive alkaline chemical called sodium carbonate, also found in dishwasher powders. Exposure to this chemical can cause adverse effects in people with sensitive skin. Even wearing the washed clothes can trigger an effect, which in some cases may be followed by an immune reaction producing an itchy rash that can spread across the body and last for several months to a year. Some sufferers claim that simply walking down a supermarket aisle stacked with boxes of biological washing powders can make them feel itchy.

SHOE POLISH may contain a solvent called nitrobenzene. As well as providing that distinctive smell, it's also a suspected human carcinogen that affects the central nervous system, producing fatigue, headache, vertigo, general weakness, and in some cases severe depression. It interacts with alcohol, so best not to polish your shoes while having a beer. Shoe polish can also contain methylene chloride, a known animal—and suspected human—carcinogen.

DRAIN CLEARER often contains the same caustic chemicals as oven cleaner—sodium hydroxide and potassium hydroxide; or sulfuric acid. All very toxic. If you can't avoid using them, follow the safety instructions religiously.

BLEACH contains sodium hypochlorite, which irritates and corrodes mucous membranes, causing pain and vomiting if swallowed. Breathing in fumes causes coughing and choking and may cause severe irritation of the respiratory tract. Go easy with the spring cleaning and perhaps wear a shower cap while you're at it—exposing the scalp to vapors containing sodium hypochlorite has been known to cause acute, toxic alopecia (baldness), as the vapor can alter the hair structure.

ALL-PURPOSE CLEANERS typically contain a scary combination of detergents, grease-cutting agents, and possibly solvents and disinfectants, plus one or more of the following: ammonia, sodium hypochlorite, trisodium phosphate, or ethylene glycol monobutyl acetate. They can cause anything from mild to extreme irritation to the skin, eyes, nose, and throat. Chronic irritation can occur after repeated use.

METAL POLISH can provoke headaches, nausea, dizziness, hallucinations, and, at extreme levels, coma, so be careful when buffing the family silver. A typical solvent in metal polish is toluene, which has been linked in human studies to reproductive and developmental disorders. Repeated high exposure during pregnancy has been associated with nervous system defects, urinary tract and gastrointestinal problems, and raised miscarriage rates. Snap on the gloves, open the windows, and don't polish very often.

AIR FRESHENER is a misnomer with bells on! Some of these products mask unwanted smells with synthetic fragrance; others work by deadening our own sense of smell. So, although the original bad smell is still there, we just can't smell it anymore. Lots of the aerosol varieties contain isobutane, butane, and propane, which may produce simple asphyxia, with symptoms such as dizziness, disorientation, headache, excitation, central nervous system depression, and anesthesia. Try opening some windows and sprinkling some essential oils around the house instead.

DISHWASHING SOAP, like all detergents, contains chemicals called surfactants, which lower the surface tension of water, making it runnier and more able to wet surfaces and clean better. They also encourage water loss from the skin, leaving it dry and irritated. More healthful vegetable-derived surfactants are easily available, but the petrochemical versions prevail because they are cheaper. Wear rubber gloves if washing by hand. If you have a dishwasher, don't touch the powder and, better still, use an eco-friendly brand.

GREEN CLEANING TIPS

Don't mix different household cleaners or solvents together. This can turn your kitchen into a dangerous chemical experiment. If you want to avoid chemical cleaners, try using the following basic, natural cleaning agents:

White vinegar. It doesn't smell and, mixed with water, it cleans windows, glass, tiles, and surfaces.

Baking soda. Mixed with water, it becomes an all-purpose cleaner for sinks and baths, and can be sprinkled over carpets as a deodorizer.

Salt. Use it for scouring pots and pans.

Lemon juice. This can be used as a bleach for laundry or, mixed with vinegar, to de-clog sinks.

Olive oil. Mix it with vinegar to polish furniture.

Choose "green" cleaning products wherever possible.

SAFE-KITCHEN CHECKLIST

■ If you use nonstick cookware, then keep temperatures low and ventilation high (see Perfluorinates, Chapter 3). Throw away the pans if there are any signs of surface degradation.

■ Use glass and ceramic food containers rather than plastics. Especially avoid storing food in direct contact with soft plastics.

■ Keep cleaning products well away from foodstuffs.

■ Don't use triclosan-impregnated cutting boards or other kitchen products.

■ Avoid having MDF or particleboard cabinets in the kitchen, if possible—especially newly installed ones. If new cabinets of this type are installed, give them a good chance to air out before putting food into your kitchen.

■ Use exhaust fans to take away smoke and cooking smells—don't use kitchen air fresheners.

■ Don't microwave in plastic.

Home Improvement Hazards

Whether you're strapping on a tool belt yourself or bringing in the professionals, home remodeling can cause a sharp spike in levels of indoor pollution. Pollution levels are typically high when the work is done and may remain high for a long time afterward, depending on the products used. There are many reasons to exercise caution while home-remodeling or decorating projects are under way, and it's best if you can seal off the areas being renovated—or temporarily move out altogether if that's an option.

■ Up to 90% of the interior surface area of a building could have a synthetic petrochemical covering or coating. These materials will commonly contain numerous defoamers, stabilizers, and various other chemicals whose effects on health are largely unknown.

Avoid using circular saws or other power tools on particleboard or MDF at home without excellent ventilation and some form of breathing protection. The best approach is to have the material cut accurately to your specs at the lumberyard. If you do cut it at home, it's best if other people aren't present at the time and that you seal all surfaces as quickly as possible to stop them off-gassing into your home. Untreated, freshly cut MDF is not a safe option in the author's opinion, unless it's a formaldehyde-free version.

Paint and other decorative finishes made from natural raw materials are a real alternative to conventional paints made from petrochemical derivatives. Natural paints are simple to use and offer high standards of protection and longevity. Because they do not contain petrochemical ingredients, they bring a number of environmental and health benefits. They are also more "breatheable" and do not attract as much dust.

Many of the synthetic solvents used in conventional paints are classified as carcinogenic, and during application their concentrations in the air can exceed recommended levels by up to seven times. As a result, professional painters are prone to suffer from dermatitis, bronchitis, asthma, and nervous system disorders. Petrochemical paint manufacturers promote their water-based paints as a less-toxic alternative to their oil-based products, but check them out thoroughly first: They may actually contain more chemicals than the oil-based type they are intended to replace. Vinyl resins, such as those found in conventional emulsion wall paints, can damage lungs, liver, and blood, and are skin irritants and possible carcinogens.

▪ Seal off-gassing sources (such as particleboard and MDF) with impermeable barriers like a heavy coating of low-VOC varnish or latex paint.

▪ Keep new furnishings and building materials in storage for a few weeks or even months before you bring them into your home. This will allow the highest levels of off-gassing to occur outside the home. If this is not possible, increase the ventilation in the affected area(s) by opening windows and doors or increasing mechanical ventilation levels for as long as possible.

▪ Buy paints, cleaners, and solvents in small quantities—just enough for what you need. Recycle old or unwanted cans and bottles and, if you can, store leftover products in separate buildings like a garage.

▪ Keep lids on tight.

On-Body Pollutants

These are the creams, lotions, and other potions that we smooth over our skin, massage into our hair, pat around our eyes, brush on our lashes, and rub on our lips; that we roll or spray under our arms, bathe in, and that some people occasionally even douche with. The average woman at her "toilette" can use twenty products or more in one sitting and may reapply some of them several times a day.

And men are catching up fast. Some really do splash it on all over—often with dubious results, going out with hair like meringue peaks and leaving a potent blend of synthetic-macho fragrance in their wake. Most generally available personal care products contain a lot of chemicals. Even ones that carry words like "organics," "fruits of the forest," or some other natural-sounding name are more likely to be fruits of the laboratory and "organic" as in organic chemistry. These

chemicals get inside us and we do not know the extent of their individual—let alone combined—action.

**Products named for the fruits of nature are more likely to be
fruits of the chemistry lab.**

■ Choose petrochemical-free products from brands such as Dr.
Hauschka, Weleda, or Burt's Bees.

■ Streamline your personal care routine to use fewer products. Start
to work on your beauty regime from the inside out too. Drink lots of
water and get plenty of fresh air and exercise!

■ Try to cut down on cosmetic use. In many cases, it's tantamount to
covering your skin in a very thin layer of plastic.

■ Avoid products that contain synthetic fragrance.

■ The cosmetics and personal-grooming industry is not regulated like
the food industry, yet a lot of the contents can be absorbed transdermally. So as you scan a contents list full of chemicals like the ones
shown on page 106, ask yourself the question: Would I eat this? And
if you wouldn't, then perhaps think twice about putting it on your
skin; the skin is the largest organ of the body and a lot of absorption
occurs through it.

■ Use caution with sunscreens; a lot of new sunscreens and some new
cosmetics contain a chemical (titanium dioxide) as an infinitesimally
small *nanoparticle*. There are concerns about this chemical's ability to
pass through the skin or be inhaled. Studies have shown that inhaled
nanoparticles can be much more toxic to health than microparticles of
the same chemical (see Chapter 6).

COMMON CHEMICALS IN PERSONAL CARE PRODUCTS

capric/caprylic triglycerides

cetearyl alcohol

cetyl alcohol

cocamide DEA

cocamidopropyl betaine

diazolidinyl urea

diethanolamine

dimethicone

emulsifying wax

FD & C colors

glyceryl stearate

imidazolidinyl urea

lanolin

mineral oils

monoethanolamine

myristamine oxide

octyl methoxycinnamate

olefin sulfonate

parabens

petrolatum

phenoxyethanol

phthalates

polyethylene glycol

polysorbate

propylene glycol

sodium lauryl sulphate

stearalkonium chloride

synthetic fragrances (musks)

tetrasodium EDTA

triclosan

triethanolamin

Note: Chemicals shown in boldface are described in Chapter 3.

In-Car Pollution

In many ways, the car is a microcosm of the home, with its leather or fabric upholstery, electrical gadgetry, lighting, carpet, phone, in-car entertainment system, and lots and lots of plastic. Almost everything you get exposed to in the home will also be in the car: flame retardants in abundance, perfluorinates to resist staining, formaldehyde in the carpets, phthalates and bisphenol A in the plastics.

So, what exactly is that new-car smell? The answer is a complex mixture of volatile organic compounds (VOCs), primarily alkanes and substituted benzenes along with a few aldehydes and ketones. Nearly every solid surface inside a vehicle is a fabric or plastic that is held together in part by various adhesives and sealers. Off-gassing of the residual solvents and other chemicals from these materials leads to a dilute mist of VOCs floating about in the passenger compartment. So before you push the air recirculation button to keep out all that nasty outdoor pollution, first consider what's already in the air inside the car.

A Japanese study revealed that the "new-car smell" could contain up to 35 times the healthful limit set for VOCs in Japanese cars in their domestic market, making it an experience akin to glue-sniffing. The chemicals found included ethyl benzene, xylene, formaldehyde, and toluene used in paints and adhesives. The study reported that it took three years for the level in cars to fall below the safe limit set for vehicles by the Japanese health ministry, a limit set in response to an increase in the number of car owners suffering from symptoms typically associated with "sick-building syndrome." Official figures are not yet available, but suffice it to say that ventilation is once again key, and sucking air through the chemically infused plastic vents is probably not as effective as just cracking open the windows.

Clearly, that new-car smell isn't good for you, and many people experience an otherwise inexplicable nausea when inside a very new car. So it's important to air it out as much as possible. It can take about six months for the new-car smell to fade and the related health risks to subside. Even if a car has off-gassed substantially, high temperatures can revitalize all those VOCs, so try not to leave the car parked in direct sunlight on a warm day. If you do, then it's good to air it out well with all the windows and doors open before you get in.

▪ A far more cost-effective and more healthful option is to buy a secondhand fuel-efficient car rather than a new one, since the chemicals will have had a chance to off-gas and the indoor pollution levels will be much lower than with a vehicle straight off the production line.

▪ Keep abreast of new products on the market, since car manufacturers are slowly getting more tuned in to making greener, cleaner machines. If you research this, you'll find that some brands will have lower chemical content than others.

▪ There are no government restrictions on in-car pollution levels. For a lot of manufacturers, the main goal is to keep the VOCs low enough to prevent fogging of the windows—without much thought given to the hazards of such high chemical concentrations in an enclosed space.

▪ Some car dealers even sell "new-car smell" fragrance sticks to keep that fresh-from-the-showroom aroma going on indefinitely!

▪ Pregnant women and young children should avoid spending extended time in brand-new cars.

▪ If you feel dizzy or slightly intoxicated while driving, pull over, get out of the car, and get some fresh air before proceeding.

Understanding that your indoor environments may be significantly polluted—and how—is the first step toward reducing your exposure to toxic chemicals. The benefits will be apparent in the short, medium, and long term, and while not many of us can afford to change all our flooring, furniture, and so on in one step, we can all improve our indoor air quality significantly just by introducing better ventilation and by keeping house dust to a minimum through regular dusting and vacuuming.

In addition, we can all streamline our list of cleaning and personal-grooming products, and be more aware of the new consumer products we introduce into our homes. Other indoor environments that we spend a lot of time in include schools, offices, and public transportation. These are places where we have far less control over our immediate environment and where much more utilitarian—and less healthful—product choices are often made. Often a lot of cheaper, more synthetic, stain- and flame-resistant building products are used. In some buildings, the toxic combinations are so bad that it is said to have "sick-building syndrome"—a phenomenon in which a high proportion of the people who work in the building experience adverse health effects such as headaches; eye, nose, or throat irritation; dry or itchy skin; dizziness; fatigue; or nausea. Changing the chemical content of these places is far more difficult than changing things at home, but the same basic solutions apply: plenty of ventilation and dust removal will help. And if you really think you or your kids are suffering from exposure to toxic chemicals at work or school, do something about it. Discuss it with fellow workers or parents, and take it up with the powers that be. No one should have to work or be educated in a significantly polluted environment.

CHAPTER 5

Rules and Regulations

"Contemporary civilization differs in one particularly distinctive feature from those which preceded it: speed. The change has come about within a generation," noted historian Marc Bloch in the 1930s. This certainly holds true for the chemical industry and its short, extraordinarily prolific history. In the West, we expect new, improved products on a weekly basis. We purchase gadgets, gizmos, and everyday items without thinking about what goes into them or where they go when we finish with them. Right behind us are new mass markets—China and India—with almost unfathomable potential demand for chemically laden consumer goods. Given the rising rates of non-infectious diseases and pervasive global contaminants, we should pass this knowledge on to developing nations and support them in creating regulatory measures that control chemicals and promote sustainability. But how do we do that, when our own regulatory systems are inconsistent and piecemeal?

Regulatory Matters

The best way to sum up the brief history of chemical legislation is to say that it has been reactive—taking action only *after* a problem has been identified. This is different from the pharmaceutical industry, where products are subject to much greater safety testing *before* they can be brought to market, and where regular updates occur as technology and medical practice evolve. Although pharmaceuticals is a far-from-perfect industry and terrible mistakes like DES and thalidomide do occur, it's still a world away from the situation we find ourselves in with chemical industry regulation.

The publication of *Silent Spring* by Rachel Carson in 1962 acted as a wake-up call to the world about the impact of synthetic chemicals on nature. Yet almost half a century later, the regulatory systems are still floundering in the face of past mistakes and a burgeoning chemical industry. Furthermore, our ability to categorically test or prove whether a chemical, alone or in combination with others, does harm or not remains elusive. Even though we now know beyond a doubt about the risks associated with POPs and PBTs, other chemicals with similar hazard profiles are still being produced in high volume and are added to products that we come into intimate contact with, without adequate testing and regulation.

This reactive approach to chemical regulation is clearly unsatisfactory, especially in light of the damning evidence against so many synthetic substances in common use. Ample evidence points to the adverse role they play in many health issues, to their sad and undeniable effects on wildlife, and to the fact that there is probably not a single place on earth uncontaminated by man-made chemicals.

There is probably not a single place on earth uncontaminated by man-made chemicals.

Many critics of big business have commented on the systemic bias toward large, global corporations when developing regulations that claim to protect the environment and public health. Although the regulatory agencies may be well-intentioned, they often fail. This is due, in part, to the "revolving door" policy, where regulatory bodies hire past and future employees of the industries they are supposed to regulate. Then there is the fact that governments are always juggling their need to protect human health and the environment with the need to encourage industry to grow and develop new products. In addition, many of the regulatory agencies do not have the funds, manpower, or legal authority needed to effectively perform their work.

Even if it were not diluted by the intense lobbying efforts of regulated industries, legislation simply would not be able to keep up with the current pace of technological change and development. For example, the U.S. Environmental Protection Agency (EPA) reviews an average of 1,700 new compounds per year—a total of nearly 32,000 since the passage of the 1976 Toxic Substances Control Act (TSCA). Of these 32,000 chemicals submitted to the EPA, most "do not include test data of any type, and only about 15 percent include health or safety test data," according to a 1995 report to Congress by the General Accounting Office (GAO). According to the report, an additional 62,000 chemicals were already in commercial use when TSCA was enacted in the late 1970s, and since then the EPA has required testing on only 200 of these "grandfathered" chemicals. In the absence of test data, the EPA evaluates toxicity of new chemicals the best they can, using mathematical models that compare new chemicals with known chemicals of similar molecular structure.

A BRIEF HISTORY OF U.S. AND GLOBAL
CHEMICAL REGULATION

1962 Rachel Carson publishes *Silent Spring*, the book that many environmentalists would argue gives the impetus that launches the modern environmental movement.

1970 The U.S. Environmental Protection Agency (EPA) is established to help protect the nation's public health and environment through research, education, and enforcement of environmental laws, including the 1970 Clean Air Act.

1972 The EPA bans the use of DDT, a widely used pesticide found to be carcinogenic and accumulating in the food chain.

1974 Congress passes the Safe Drinking Water Act, setting health-based standards for the quality of the public water supply.

1976 Congress passes the Toxic Substances Control Act (TSCA), originally intended to assure the safety of new and existing chemicals, and to make information provided by chemical companies available to the public. Under the law, the EPA starts to review chemicals in 1979.

1977 The Consumer Products Safety Commission (CPSC) bans the fire retardant tris from use in children's sleepwear after it was shown to be a potent animal carcinogen.

1979 The EPA bans PCBs and two herbicides containing dioxins, setting the stage for the phaseout of all dioxin manufacturing and use in the U.S.

1983 The Report of the UN Brundtland Commission illustrates the global concern for the state of the environment and popularizes the phrase "sustainable development." This is defined in the report as a way "to meet the needs of the present without compromising the ability of future generations to meet their own needs."

1988 The EPA bans the pesticide chlordane, used to treat over 30 million U.S. homes since the 1950s. Chlordane has been linked to

(continued)

(*A Brief History of U.S. and Global Chemical Regulation* continued)

childhood and adult cancers and a wide variety of respiratory and neurological disorders.

1989 The EPA bans commercial use of asbestos, but the decision is overturned by a federal appeals court in 1991. Since this time, no chemicals have been banned in the U.S.

1992 The UN convenes the Rio Earth Summit. The largest environmental conference held up to this date, the summit draws over 30,000 people, including more than 100 heads of state. The summit's "Declaration on Environment and Development" addresses the environmentally sound management of toxic chemicals, including the illegal international traffic in toxic and dangerous products. Additionally, the declaration states: "In order to protect the environment, the precautionary approach shall be widely applied by states according to their capabilities. Where there are threats of serious or irreversible damage, lack of full scientific certainty shall not be used as a reason for postponing cost-effective measures to prevent environmental degradation." This establishes the first legal precedent for the "Precautionary Principle," giving the environment the benefit of the doubt over unsustainable development.

2001 The UN adopts the Stockholm Convention on Persistent Organic Pollutants (POPs). Signatories agree to phase out and limit production of 12 major POPs—toxic, bioaccumulative chemicals that can cause biological havoc. At present, over 140 countries have ratified the Convention. The U.S. has signed it, but has not yet ratified it.

2003 The European Commission proposes REACH, a new regulatory framework for the Registration, Evaluation and Authorisation of Chemicals throughout Europe. Unlike U.S. law, REACH places the burden of proof on the manufacturer to demonstrate that chemicals are safe before they are placed on the market. REACH was formally adopted by the EU in 2006 and went into force in mid-2007.

Chemical Regulation in the U.S.

Chemicals in our water, food, cosmetics, and consumer goods are regulated by a patchwork of laws and governmental bodies at the state and federal level. What nearly all these regulations have in common is a failure to adequately test most chemicals before they are introduced to the marketplace. In most instances, serious harm must be demonstrated before regulators get involved. And even then, the burden of proof is on the individuals harmed or the government agency to prove that a chemical is dangerous, not on the manufacturer to prove it is safe. Because cancer often takes 20 or more years to develop and may be caused by the interaction of multiple chemicals, proving a causal link under current law is difficult and expensive. For example, EPA's asbestos ban in 1989 was overturned two years later by a federal appeals court on the grounds that the EPA had not sufficiently proved that the ban was necessary to protect human health. That was the last chemical banned by the federal agency.

Following is a brief overview of the main regulatory bodies in the U.S. responsible for keeping our food, water, cosmetics, and consumer products safe and effective.

The U.S. Environmental Protection Agency (EPA)

Founded in 1970, the EPA is the main governmental body charged with protecting public health and the environment. There is no doubt that the EPA has accomplished a lot over the past decades. Without the efforts of the EPA, our water supplies, air quality, and general environment would be far more degraded than they are. The EPA's record on controlling chemicals in consumer goods, however, is more questionable.

The EPA regulates the manufacture of commercial chemicals

through the 1976 Toxic Substances Control Act (TSCA). When the EPA started reviewing chemicals under the law in 1979, over 60,000 chemicals were "grandfathered" in. These were considered safe unless the EPA could prove an "unreasonable risk" to human health or the environment and demonstrate that the benefits of a ban or restriction outweighed the risks. The costly and time-consuming burden of obtaining the necessary data has been on the EPA. Since the law was enacted, the EPA has sought health information on less than 200 of these pre-existing commercial chemicals, accounting for an estimated 99% of chemicals now in commercial use, and has banned or restricted only 5 of these chemicals or chemical groups!

A different standard applies to the roughly 32,000 "new" compounds introduced since 1979, of which the EPA has approved 90% without restrictions. To impose restrictions on new chemicals, the EPA must demonstrate evidence of potential harm, which is difficult since the law requires very limited data from manufacturers and does not require them to do testing. In the absence of data, the EPA relies on computer modeling and comparisons to other chemicals to determine risk. According to a 1995 report by the General Accounting Office (GAO), the EPA has received health information on only 15% of the 32,000 new compounds. And what little information exists is often kept from the public due to manufacturers' claims of confidentiality allowed by the law.

Critics of the agency claim that the EPA and the public are still much in the dark regarding the health impact of the vast majority of chemicals used in everyday products. In an effort to get better information within the framework of current law, in 1998 the EPA launched the voluntary High Production Volume (HPV) Challenge, with the goal of obtaining basic "screening-level" toxicity data on the approximately 28,000 chemicals produced at rates of over 1 million pounds per year, and making the data publicly available. While the program has been helpful, its impact has been limited by its voluntary status. The group Environmental Defense points out in its 2004 Status Report on the program that over 500 of the original list of chemicals have either been withdrawn or exempted from the program, while over 700 new chemicals have been added to the HPV list but are not officially covered by the program.

The EPA has been successful in removing some of the worst toxic chemicals from the marketplace—including PCBs, dioxin, and the pesticides DDT and chlordane—and has placed some restrictions on over 3,000 "new" chemicals. And through the Clean Air Act, it has been responsible for a significant reduction in VOCs in paints, adhesives, and similar products. Yet the vast majority of chemicals in use today have escaped their scrutiny. Under current law, the EPA does not appear to have the authority or the budget to adequately safeguard the public from the risks of hazardous chemicals.

The Food and Drug Administration (FDA)

The oldest consumer protection agency in the U.S., the FDA is responsible for protecting public health by assuring the safety and effectiveness of human and veterinary drugs, medical devices, the nation's food supply, and cosmetics. Under FDA rules, cosmetics include all articles "intended to be rubbed, poured, sprinkled, sprayed on, introduced into, or otherwise applied to the human body . . . for cleansing, beautifying, promoting attractiveness, or altering the appearance" (FD&C Act, Sec. 201). This definition includes products such as moisturizers, makeup, perfumes, lipsticks, fingernail polish, shampoos, hairsprays and colorants, toothpaste, and deodorants, as well as any ingredients used in these products. The same law defines "drugs" as articles "intended for use in the diagnosis, cure, mitigation, treatment, or prevention of disease . . . and articles intended to affect the structure or any function of the body of man or other animals." A number of products, such as antidandruff shampoos, toothpastes with fluoride, or deodorants with antiperspirants, are considered by the FDA to be both cosmetics and drugs and must, therefore, comply with the requirements of both.

The main difference between regulations for cosmetics and drugs is that all drugs, whether prescription or over-the-counter, need pre-approval from the FDA before being put on the market. To be approved for sale, an over-the-counter drug must either comply with established standards for "safe and effective" products or the manufacturer must provide adequate test data. Cosmetics, on the other hand, are essentially self-regulated—it is the manufacturer's responsibility to assure that its cosmetic products and ingredients are safe and properly labeled. With the exception of color additives, they do not have to comply with any specific safety requirements. It is up to individual cosmetics manufacturers to determine the safety of their products, as they define safety, typically relying on patch tests to make sure that the product does not irritate skin.

FDA regulations do prohibit the sale of "adulterated" products that contain ingredients known to be "poisonous or deleterious" under normal use, and the agency has banned the use of several compounds, including bithinol, mercury, and some carcinogens such as chloroform and methylene chloride. Still, many questionable chemicals—including phthalates, formaldehyde, and coal tar—are allowed under current FDA guidelines.

Many questionable chemicals—including phthalates, formaldehyde, and coal tar—are allowed in cosmetics under current FDA guidelines.

While the cosmetics industry has a generally good track record for product safety, critics charge that trace amounts of hazardous and endocrine-disrupting chemicals—including phthalates, lead acetate (in hair coloring), and dioxane (in baby shampoo)—are absorbed into the body and can cause harm: if not immediately, then over time from cumulative exposure. In response to such health concerns, California enacted the California Safe Cosmetics Act in 2007, mandating that manufacturers notify health authorities if cosmetics contain any potentially hazardous ingredients. In Europe, cosmetics are now regulated under REACH, requiring manufacturers to meet stringent requirements for health and environmental impact.

In the absence of strong manufacturing controls, accurate and complete labeling is especially important to consumers. While it's true that all drugs, cosmetics, and packaged foods must follow strict labeling requirements in the U.S., some loopholes exist. In general, all ingredients of packaged foods and cosmetics must be listed in descending order of quantity. Exempted from labeling requirements in packaged foods are any "indirect additives" (including pesticide residues). Indirect food additives are those that migrate into the food in trace amounts due to its packaging, storage, or handling, including an estimated 2,000 materials and coatings used in food packaging. The FDA is charged with enforcing pesticide tolerances on most food products and with overseeing the safety of both indirect additives and direct additives such as preservatives, flavors, and colors. While the agency is credited with doing a diligent job of sorting through the thousands of pages of data supporting the safety of various food additives, it is questionable whether adequate testing is done with packaging materials and coatings, which may enter foods unintentionally.

WHAT'S IN A LABEL—AND WHAT'S NOT?

Foods, drugs, and cosmetics all must follow strict labeling requirements established by the U.S. Food and Drug Administration (FDA). In general, all food, drugs, and cosmetics must list all ingredients in descending order of quantity. Products that are considered both cosmetics and drugs must list the drug components separately as "active ingredients." Food producers are required to list all "direct" additives, including preservatives, flavor enhancers, and artificial colors. Certain items, such as natural colors, may be listed under generic terms, such as "colorings." New regulations also require producers to list common food allergens in simple terms like "contains milk," rather than requiring the reader to understand more technical terms like "casein."

What's **not** listed on food labels are so-called "indirect" additives. These include a variety of materials—including pesticide residues—that may become part of the food in trace amounts due to its handling, storage, or leaching from the packaging. With cosmetics, the law allows manufacturers to use the terms "flavor" (in toothpaste, for example) and "fragrance" to cover all ingredients used for those purposes. Labels do not need to list their component chemicals separately, even though fragrances often contain phthalates and synthetic musks and may contain any of up to a hundred other chemicals. Other food ingredients may be exempted from labeling by the FDA for confidentiality purposes and listed as "other ingredients." Cosmetics may also contain chemical by-products or contaminants not listed on the label. For example, researchers have recently found phthalates in 8 common consumer fragrances, and others found dioxane, a possible human carcinogen, in 15 popular baby shampoos. Accurate labeling of cosmetics is the responsibility of the manufacturer, and labels are not pre-approved by the FDA, so the buyer should beware.

The Consumer Products Safety Commission

The U.S. Consumer Product Safety Commission (CPSC) is a small federal regulatory agency created in 1972 to protect the public from unreasonable risks of injury and death from fire, electrical, chemical, or mechanical hazards associated with some 15,000 types of consumer products—everything from baby teethers to stepladders and microwave ovens. In addition to providing safety information, the CPSC has the power to develop mandatory standards, to recall dangerous products, and to restrict or ban hazardous products when they believe that no standard would adequately protect the public. For example, in 1977 the CPSC banned the fire retardant tris from use in children's sleepwear after it was determined that the chemical was a powerful animal carcinogen.

Chemical-related bans by CPSC are fairly rare. In addition to tris in pajamas, CPSC has banned candles with lead-core wicks, certain flammable adhesives, some asbestos-based products, and formaldehyde foam building insulation (later reversed).

Short of banning products, the CPSC may issue warnings and recommendations. For example, in 1998 the CPSC was petitioned to ban children's teethers and chew toys containing the plasticizer diisononyl phthalate (DINP). Based on a review of the relevant health data, the CPSC did not impose a ban but requested industry to remove phthalates from soft rattles and teethers "as a precaution while more scientific work is done." CPSC also set an acceptable daily intake level for DINP, setting it at "100 times less than the amount found not to cause any adverse health effects in laboratory animals." The safety of phthalates remains controversial, and both Japan and the European Union currently have bans in place on the use of some phthalates in children's mouthing toys.

Like other agencies, CPSC reacts to problems only after they occur and has banned chemical uses in only a handful of cases. Because CPSC does not certify products as safe, the lack of a recall or warning cannot be taken as an assurance of safety. That responsibility is shared by the manufacturer and the consumer. Also, consumer products, such as fabrics, are not required to carry labels listing ingredients such as chemical treatments and coatings, making it difficult to make informed decisions.

Global Regulations: The Stockholm Convention

In 2001, the United Nations completed negotiations on the Stockholm Convention on Persistent Organic Pollutants (POPs), which went into force in 2004. The Stockholm Convention is one of the major achievements in global chemical regulation; it followed directly from principles established at the UN's 1992 Rio Earth Summit. Signatories agreed to ban or strictly limit the production and use of 12 of the worst persistent organic pollutants (POPs), known as the "dirty dozen." These toxic chemicals—many used as pesticides—are known to bioaccumulate in the world's food web, harming human health and the environment. Over 140 countries have ratified the international treaty to date. The U.S. has signed and expressed support for the Convention, but has yet to ratify the treaty—a step that would require congressional approval and changes to the U.S. laws governing pesticides and industrial chemicals.

The treaty also outlined key principles for a less toxic world, including the prevention of new toxic, persistent, and bioaccumulative chemicals; reduction of existing ones; and substitution with less dangerous alternatives. At present, however, the Stockholm Treaty covers only 12 chemicals: 9 pesticides, polychlorinated biphenyls (PCBs), and the industrial by-products dioxins and furans. Brominated flame retardants and perfluorinates are up for consideration for POP status—if this were to occur, it would mean radical changes for the chemical industry.

The UN should be commended for the POPs Convention, as should all nations that played a key role and made sure that it came to fruition. But the Convention only addresses 12 compounds, many of which had already been banned since the 1970s in developed nations like Great Britain, other European nations, the U.S., and Canada. A more skeptical view would be: What took responsible governments so long, nearly 40 years, to try to implement global controls on such damaging substances? And what about the rest of the chemicals that are manufactured, traded, and used in consumer products? In the European Union, this number is believed to be about 30,000 chemicals. How well are those being regulated? The answer is: Very poorly.

REACH—The European Solution

Not only has the U.S. tried and failed to adequately regulate chemicals, so too has the European Union. While both have tried to implement more stringent testing on new chemicals coming onto the market, older substances are still allowed to be used despite little or no safety data. That "burden of the past"—all those existing substances about which we know so little—is of great concern. Any responsible society would prohibit the use of a chemical until it was well tested and proven safe for humans and wildlife.

Industry's response has been very different. Its message is along the lines of: We've used these chemicals for decades with no obvious adverse effects, so let's continue using them without testing. But, as this book reveals, such confidence is misplaced. How can the manufacturer of a chemical or compound, without adequate testing, convince you, the consumer, that their substance is not a contributing factor in decreasing fertility, the rising number of birth defects, or higher incidences of diabetes and various cancers? We know that certain diseases are increasing, but without good data on the health effects of chemicals, we cannot say why.

It is against this global backdrop that the European Union (EU) decided that a completely new approach to chemical regulation was needed. In 1998, when the United Kingdom held the presidency of the EU, it said that new chemical legislation should:

- address the knowledge gap on the tens of thousands of substances already on the market in consumer products to which humans, wildlife, and the wider environment are constantly exposed; and

- reverse the burden of proof to require that chemical companies do sufficient testing to make sure that a chemical is safe before it goes on the market—rather than make it the regulator's responsibility to prove harm.

Following from this, the EU Commission wrote the "Chemicals White Paper," leading to the creation of a new regulatory framework for chemicals, called REACH: the Regulation, Evaluation and Authorisation of Chemicals. REACH proposed a major new system to test a large number of chemicals for their effects on human health and the environment. This would, for the first time, provide adequate safety data on the chemicals that we have been using "blind" for decades, plus would completely reverse the burden of proof so that "no data, no market" would be the rule. If a company doesn't have the data to prove that a chemical it produces is safe, then it will be removed from the market.

The key aim of REACH is to protect humans, wildlife, and the environment from chemical harm while not undermining the competitiveness of EU chemical manufacturing. From a consumer's point of view, the key elements in REACH, if enforced (see box), *should* protect the public and the wider environment.

THE KEY ELEMENTS OF REACH

- To stop the use of chemicals that are of very high concern: This includes chemicals that are persistent, bioaccumulative, and toxic (PBTs), very persistent and very bioaccumulative VPVBs, and endocrine-disrupting chemicals (EDCs), where human, wildlife, or wider environmental exposure can occur.

- Substitution: Chemicals that contaminate the environment should be replaced with safer, less toxic alternatives.

- The right to know (RTK): Manufacturers and consumers have a right to know which chemicals are in what products.

- Reversal of the burden of proof: Manufacturers and distributors must prove that a chemical is safe, rather than regulators needing to prove harm.

- No data, no market: If a manufacturer does not have the safety data for a chemical, it should not be used in consumer products.

Will it REACH where other legislation has failed?

After much negotiation, the REACH regulation was formally adopted by the EU in December 2006 and went into force on June 1, 2007. In its first incarnation, the REACH proposal was expected to make dramatic improvements to chemical industry legislation and to cause a major shakeup in accountability, leading to extensive testing on 30,000 economically traded chemicals in the EU. The EU predicted that the successful implementation of REACH would bring savings in health care of over 50 billion euros over a 30-year period.

However, after what some EU officials claim to be the biggest lobbying effort they have ever seen, from European and American chemical manufacturers, the testing requirements have been diluted and further loopholes are expected to be added under the intense lobbying pressure. In addition, the U.S. government has criticized REACH for hampering global trade. Particularly troubling is the section of the law addressing EDCs. How much proof will be needed before countries within the EU stop the most vulnerable members of our society (babies and children) from being exposed to such worrisome chemicals? Many people object to this deep involvement of lobbyists and think it's time for the EU to start regulating the lobbyists.

In its original form, REACH legislation was predicted to bring health-care savings of over 50 billion euros over 30 years.

So What Can We Expect?

Reducing our dependence on common toxic chemicals requires a combination of factors, ideally all working together at the same time. These include:

- strong laws requiring chemical companies to be responsible for their products' effects on health and the environment, and
- greater public awareness and consumer participation in the demand for toxic-free products and processes.

In the absence of strong chemical safety laws, accurate product labeling is especially important, since this is vital to the public's right-to-know about toxic materials used in consumer products. This knowledge enables consumers to refuse to buy products containing particular toxic chemicals. Labeling systems are already in use for a number of products, including PVC-free toys, mercury-free thermometers, organically grown cotton T-shirts, and chlorine-free bleached paper.

In the short term, probably the best we can realistically expect is better labeling and the gradual phasing out of known PBT chemicals. What we cannot expect is a precautionary approach to be suddenly adopted by an industry that has gone unchecked and virtually unregulated for so many decades. The REACH legislation exemplifies the ways in which lobbying has become a refined, behind-closed-doors political tool, allowing big business to put its interest in maximizing profits ahead of people's health.

Without wanting to paint too dark a picture, the reality is that the chance of the industry pulling itself up by its green bootstraps in the near future, without intense consumer and regulatory pressure, is a long shot. While regulatory attempts are admirable and every step forward should be acknowledged and applauded, the overriding concern is that enforcing any regulation on such a disparate, prolific, and powerful industry takes a long and sustained effort.

To motivate us to action, it should be enough to know that nearly every pregnant and lactating woman on the earth today will, often unwittingly and certainly unwillingly, be exposing her unborn or newborn child to a variety of chemicals. Many of these are known to be toxic—and the health effects of many remain unknown—and there's not a thing she can do about it. This is unacceptable in any civilized society, and as consumers we must stop blindsiding ourselves. We must ask: What makes this fabric "crease-proof," this cleaner "super-powered," this carpet "stain-proof"? What mass of plastic, electronics, and chemicals am I adding to global toxic waste every time I upgrade my phone, iPod, laptop, car, etc.? Most important, what effect is all our ignorance having on our children? We are all living in debt, in more ways than one.

CHAPTER 6

Hope and Risks for the Future

Much health and fitness literature feeds us the idea that we can de-tox, re-tox, and then de-tox again—almost ad infinitum and at will. To a limited extent, it's true that a period of healthful eating, exercise, and staying off alcohol, drugs, and cigarettes will allow the body time to expel accumulated toxicity—particularly with respect to many of the things that we do knowingly and consensually. However, as we have seen, when it comes to certain classes of toxic chemicals, the "pollution" of our bodies can be very long-term and almost irreversible. With cruel irony, it can be argued that, short of having a baby, it's very difficult to reduce the PBT chemicals that accumulate in our tissues.

Novel molecular configurations lining our frying pans might offer new ways to cook our eggs, but unfortunately we now have to ask ourselves: What's in the egg I'm frying, what was in the chicken that laid the egg, and what's in the pan it's frying in? It might be the case that the chemical that makes frying your eggs easier could react with a chemical that has already bioaccumulated in the egg itself. When you eat the egg, it might bioaccumulate in you and potentially harm your reproductive system, your own eggs or sperm. You could then pass this on to your offspring—and the old story about the chicken and the egg could start to take on a new and much more sinister meaning.

Another ominous upshot, from research on endocrine-disrupting chemicals, indicates that they seem to be hitting the male of the species particularly hard, and specifically in their reproductive systems. The combination of higher incidences of reproductive-system birth defects in baby boys, lower sperm counts, and rising cases of testicular cancer among young men could mean a gradual loss of our ability to reproduce as a species—perhaps an insidious form of natural selection with a chemical twist. Who knows?

The combination of higher incidences of reproductive-system birth defects in baby boys, lower sperm counts, and rising cases of testicular cancer among young men could mean a gradual loss of our ability to reproduce as a species.

What we do know is that we need sustainable or greener chemistry to be the rule, not the exception. Adopting a precautionary policy when it comes to using both new and old synthetic chemicals in consumer products is the only sensible way forward. We must give infants and children the benefit of the doubt and ensure that adequate testing is done, rather than continue the everyday use of chemicals that we know so little about.

"But, wait," chimes the chorus of chemical companies, corporations, and complacent consumers. "We are all living longer, so what's the big fuss about?" Well, firstly, "we" is a very general term, and while a lot of us are living longer, it is often with various complaints that were uncommon fifty years ago. Also, the problems posed by toxic chemicals are often more far-reaching and subtle than life-threatening conditions. It's about disruption of human and animal behavior and the undermining basic human right to fulfill one's potential without attention deficit disorders, neurological impairments, messed-up hormones, or the psychosexual burden of being born with a sexually ambiguous or deformed reproductive system.

Take endocrine-disrupting chemicals alone. Hormones are the natural chemical messengers of life on earth: They tell squirrels when to hibernate and salmon when to swim upriver to spawn. They control when women ovulate, plus myriad other essential human functions. They are present in the blood in minuscule concentrations, often for only short periods of time, and yet have powerful effects on us. Witness mood-swinging adolescence, the power of adrenaline, sexual desire, PMS and male aggression. It's hard enough keeping ourselves in check without fake messages flooding our hormonal systems. But as we've seen, many synthesized chemicals have been shown to be good imitators of our natural hormones, and some can actually interfere with this delicate, powerful, complex, and intensely interrelated system. There is plenty of evidence of strange things afoot in wildlife—aquatic, avian, and terrestrial—and since what we do to the animals, we ultimately do to ourselves, the unavoidable and distinctly unpalatable truth is that it may already be happening to us. One has to ask oneself: How serious do things have to get before we collectively take action?

The sort of risk assessment done for chemicals added to everyday products is not one you would choose for yourself or those dependent on you. Would you say to yourself: I'll keep using this cream on my baby until it is proven to give my child a persistent behavioral disorder that may well affect her or his educational potential and social development? Of course not; you'd choose an alternative that you know is safe until the cream has been proven to have no short-, mid-, or long-term effects.

So, before you pop out for a few cocktails, think about the one you are slathering, massaging, slicking, and spraying onto all the different parts of your body. The shampoos, body washes, nail polishes, lipsticks, face creams, perfumes, aftershaves, shaving gels, hair gels, sprays, mousses—you've probably got a wide range of products. None of us wants to look like our personal care regime consists of a scrap of harsh soap and a rough towel, but we assure you, you *can* be pampered, soothed, and primped *without* poisoning yourself. Just choose products that don't have petroleum by-products in them, and choose greener, cleaner options—ideally without parabens, formaldehyde, phthalates, and so forth. Chemical solutions for mass-market consumer products are generally designed to make easy living cheap, but there may be a heavy personal cost as well as the obvious environmental one. If you thought that the synthetic musk in your aftershave might lower your sperm count, how attractive would it make you feel as you splashed it all over?

One major problem in all this is linking exposure to specific chemicals with specific illnesses because of the multiplicity of influences we are exposed to in contemporary life—let alone linking specific chemicals to effects on IQ, behavior, or immune-system function. Yet where specific and tragic chemical accidents have occurred, there have been clear consequences on local populations—or, in the case of DES, on the offspring of the women who were prescribed it. This is all very compelling evidence for the precautionary approach to chemicals, because laws take a long time to come into force. Look how long it took to make the case for cigarettes and cancer. Even with clear evidence, people are still unwillingly, passively exposed to cigarette smoke in many states, and it is still legal in some settings for adults to smoke where children are present.

The issue of synthetic chemicals, given their sheer quantity and ubiquity in consumer products, at first seems insurmountable. However, it has largely been a lack of scientific knowledge that has permitted such widespread use of these untested chemicals to have proceeded in the past with so little constraint and caution. The tobacco industry had the advantage of addicted consumers who simply didn't want to admit that their habits could be the agents of their own deterioration. No one, as far as we know, is addicted to any of the toxic chemicals written about in this book. While some of us might be reluctant to part company with the promise of the '50s advertising slogan "Better things for better living . . . through chemistry," in the face of what's really at stake—the legacy that we leave to our children and grandchildren—the attachment to chemical convenience seems reckless.

Although we often don't, we should all think about the broader and longer-term consequences of how we live. The phenomenon of global distillation (whereby the global winds of the world blow outward from the hot equator to the two polar cold environments), combined with the near-indestructible persistence of certain toxic chemicals, means that many of the latter end up settling in the two far poles of the world. Thirty years ago, the most surprising fact known about the polar bear was that it could be quite aggressive—but now, sadly, it is that it is one of the most toxic animals on earth, despite living far away from the industries that produce the substances that contaminate it. This is true of hundreds of contaminated animal populations, from fish to herring gulls, from frogs to whales—and, ultimately, us.

There has to be a fundamental paradigm shift in the way we live with chemicals, especially now as the dawn of nanotechnology brings with it a new type of potentially even more invasive agent—in the form of new nanotoxic substances where smaller particles of previously harmless substances start to make it to places they've never been before.

Nanomaterials and Nanoparticles

" The prospects for using engineered nanomaterials in industrial applications, medical imaging, disease diagnoses, drug delivery, cancer treatment, gene therapy, and other areas have progressed rapidly. . . . The possible toxic health effects of these nanoparticles associated with human exposure are unknown. Many fine particles generally considered 'nuisance dusts' are likely to acquire unique surface properties when engineered to nanosize and may exhibit toxic biological effects. "

Maureen R. Gwinn and Val Vallyathan, National Institute for Occupational Safety and Health, Morgantown, WV (*Environmental Health Perspectives,* Dec. 2006)

Nanoparticles are tiny (less than 100 billionths of a meter across, or about 1/1,000 the thickness of a human hair), and are already used in products as diverse as anti-aging creams, sunscreens, anti-bacterial socks, and tennis racquets. They are touted as "miracle molecules," and nanotechnology is increasingly used in new pharmaceuticals and medical applications. For example, the headline-grabbing breast-cancer drug Herceptin has a nanosized antibody that can infiltrate the HER 2 receptors of tumor cells and tell them to stop growing. The potential for nanotechnology to help treat cancer and other medical conditions is clearly very exciting. Their use in sunscreens and cosmetics, on the other hand, is arguably quite superfluous in light of early research indicating that certain nanoparticle chemicals can be very toxic, especially when in water (shown to cause rapid-onset brain damage in fish and to kill water fleas living in water contaminated with "buckyballs"—a particular kind of nanoparticle). Since many nanoparticles can cross the blood/brain barrier in humans, precaution is, you might say, a no-brainer. If any doubt exists over their potential toxicity to the environment, to wildlife, and to us, then a lot more research must be done before the chemical industry is allowed to imbue a wide range of "new and improved" consumer products with new unknown risks. The market for nanoparticles appears to be increasing rapaciously, and yet neither government regulations nor labeling requirements currently exist in any country.

We're the generation that has probably seen the greatest degree of technological change, and sometimes it's hard to know if we're waving or drowning. We appreciate the benefits some chemicals offer, but at the same time, we know beyond doubt that irreversible damage is being done to the earth's ecosystems. While we might make personal decisions to drive our cars less or stop smoking, our planet is still smoldering in front of our eyes. We know exactly how to change the ways of the world for a sustainable future, but we don't. It's an appalling lack of environmental responsibility, fueled by litigious corporations and a consumer culture based on ease and disposability.

We know exactly how to change the ways of the world for a sustainable future, but we don't.

There is no apparent limit to human invention, and it is only natural to want to drive new cars, take foreign vacations, and use cell phones, but we need to rethink collectively how to do this so that we can behave more sustainably. Against this background, self-education is essential—keeping our heads in the sand is no longer an option. It is our personal viewpoint that, once people know a little bit about the many chemicals used in everyday consumer products, they will see that their only sensible choice is to try to avoid them. We do. It might appear daunting at first, but with some simple changes to our everyday routines, it is possible to dramatically reduce exposure to common toxic chemicals. And consumers have power—so challenge your retailers, product manufacturers, and representatives in Congress. Ask questions and demand answers!

Product Guides

HOME FURNISHINGS & APPLIANCES

Sources	Chemicals of Concern	Healthful Alternatives
Synthetic carpets	Formaldehyde, other VOCs, BFRs	Choose natural fibers or carpeting certified with Green Label.
Sofas, curtains, soft furnishings	BFRs, PCFs	Choose tightly woven natural fabrics. Don't have fabrics treated with stain repellents.
Permanent-press draperies	formaldehyde	Choose non-treated fabrics.
Vinyl shower curtains	phthalates	Choose alternative materials, or air out well before using.
Consumer electronics (computers, cell phones, etc.)	BFRs, BPA	Choose items with non-plastic casings. Buy from manufacturers offering non-toxic casings. Unplug devices when not in use.
Refrigerator shelving	PBA	Use glass, not plastic.
Air fresheners, fragranced items	synthetic musk	Use small quantities of essential oils, if desired.
Floor waxes	PCFs	Use no-wax floor coverings.

Abbreviations: BPA (bisphenol A), BRF (brominated flame retardants), PCF (perfluorinates), VOC (volatile organic compound)

BUILDING MATERIALS

Sources	Chemicals of Concern	Healthful Alternatives
Kitchen/bath cabinets	formaldehyde (particleboard or MDF)	Avoid cabinets made of particleboard or MDF. Or make sure all surfaces are well sealed with a laminate or heavy coating.
Vinyl (PVC) flooring	phthalates, BPA, organotins	Use solid wood or other natural floorings.
Particleboard, MDF	formaldehyde	Choose exterior-grade plywood or certified low-emitting particleboard or low-emitting MDF.
Decorative plywood paneling	formaldehyde	Avoid interior-grade plywood paneling. Use an alternate product.
Conventional paints and varnishes	formaldehyde, BPA, organotins, toluene	Choose low-VOC or non-toxic paints and finishes.

Abbreviations: BPA (bisphenol A), MDF (medium-density fiberboard)

CLOTHING & PERSONAL CARE PRODUCTS

Sources	Chemicals of Concern	Healthful Alternatives
Cosmetics	phthalates, synthetic musk, parabens, nonylphenol, toluene	Choose simple emollients and natural non-toxic product lines. Use fewer products.
Perfumes, scented products	synthetic musk, toluene	Choose natural, non-toxic products.
Nail products	parabens, toluene	Choose natural, non-toxic products.
Shampoos, liquid soaps	phthalates, parabens, formaldehyde, synthetic musk, nonylphenol, SLS, MIT	Choose natural, non-toxic products.
Eyeglass lenses	BPA	Avoid polycarbonate lenses.

(Clothing & Personal Care Products continued)

Dental sealants	BPA	Avoid white fillings at dentist.
Toothpaste, mouthwash	formaldehyde, synthetic musk, triclosan, SLS	Choose natural, non-toxic alternatives,
Foot-care products	triclosan	Choose natural, non-toxic alternatives.
Deodorants	synthetic musk, parabens, triclosan	Choose natural, non-toxic alternatives.
Condoms	parabens	Choose other methods of birth control.
Clothes detergents, conditioners	synthetic musk	Use unscented products.
No-iron clothing, fabrics	PFCs	Choose untreated fabrics.
Heat-transfer printing (e.g., on T-shirts)	organotins	Avoid heat-transfer prints.
Waterproof clothing, footwear	PFCs	Check labels for chemicals like Teflon.
Shoe polish	toluene	Use only in well-ventilated areas.
Dry-cleaned clothing	perchloroethylene (perc)	Avoid clothing that requires dry-cleaning, or use non-perc methods.

Abbreviations: BPA (bisphenol A), PFC (perfluorinates), MIT (methylisothiazolinone), SLS (sodium lauryl sulphate)

BABY & CHILD CARE

Sources	Chemicals of Concern	Healthful Alternatives
Disposable diapers	organotins	Use cloth diapers or eco-friendly disposables.
Pajamas and other clothes	BFRs	Choose untreated fabrics.
Children's socks	organotins, triclosan	Avoid clothing with added fungicides.

Children's underwear, school uniforms, bedclothes	triclosan	Avoid anti-bacterial clothing and bedding.
Plastic feeding bottles	BPA	Use glass bottles, or discard plastic bottles every three months.
Pacifiers	phthalates	Choose natural materials or phthalate-free plastics.
Plastic toys	phthalates, triclosan	Choose natural materials or phthalate-free plastics.
Inflatable toys	phthalates, organotins	Avoid these, or use phthalate-free materials.
Baby lotions	parabens	Choose natural, non-toxic products.
Bubble bath	formaldehyde, SLS	Choose natural, non-toxic products.
Gel-like play materials	parabens	Avoid these materials unless proven non-toxic.

Abbreviations: BFR (brominated flame retardant), BPA (bisphenol A), SLS (sodium lauryl sulphate)

FOOD & COOKING EQUIPMENT

Sources	Chemicals of Concern	Healthful Alternatives
Nonstick cookware	PFCs	Use stainless-steel, cast-iron, ceramic, or porcelain enamel cookware.
Plastic cutting boards	triclosan	Choose wooden cutting boards.
Plastic food containers, plastic wrap	Phthalates, BPA	Avoid plastic food containers, wrap. Do not microwave in plastic.
Microwave popcorn	PFCs	Do not use.
Fast-food packaging	PFCs	Avoid packaged fast food, especially high-fat foods.
Water bottles	BPA	Avoid plastic water bottles, especially for repeated use.

(Food & Cooking Equipment continued)		
Food cans/containers	BPA	Minimize use of canned food, especially high-fat products.
Plastic plates, cups, utensils	BPA, triclosan	Use paper plates and cups, metal utensils for picnics.
Aspartame	formaldehyde (a by-product when it breaks down)	Avoid products with artificial sweeteners.

Abbreviations: BPA (bisphenol A), BRF (brominated flame retardants), PFC (perfluorinates), VOC (volatile organic compound)

Glossary

Additive effect: The combined effect of two or more chemicals.

Bioaccumulation: If an organism takes on a chemical at a faster rate than it can eliminate it, the chemical will accumulate in the organism. For example, PCBs tend to bind to fatty tissues in fish, accumulating in the fish and whatever eats them.

Biomagnification: The more rapid buildup of persistent, bioaccumulative toxic chemicals in animals higher up the food chain. At the top of the food chain, tissue concentrations can be millions of times higher than in the general environment.

Cocktail effect: See *Additive effect*.

Dose-response curve: A graph showing the relationship between the level of exposure to a chemical or drug and the effect on an organism. New models take into account the *timing* of the exposure as well as the amount—for example, the same dose may have a greater effect on a developing fetus or infant than on an adult.

Endocrine-disrupting chemical (EDC): These interfere with the endocrine or hormonal system, the body's own chemical messaging system, which regulates key bodily functions such as metabolism, sexual development, and growth.

Leach: To migrate from a material into the environment. For example, some chemicals that are used to coat the inside of food packaging can leach into the food. The chemical that migrates this way is a *leachate.*

Lipophilic: Literally means lipid-loving or fat-loving. Lipophilic chemicals don't readily dissolve in water, making them difficult to metabolize. They tend to remain in an animal's fatty tissues, including those in the blood, brain, and liver. If lipophilic chemicals are also *persistent,* they will tend to bioaccumulate.

Medium-density fiberboard (MDF): A significant source of formaldehyde emissions (off-gassing), along with particleboard and interior grades of plywood and wood paneling. MDF is widely used as the core material in veneered shelving, cabinets, and furniture.

Multiple chemical sensitivity (MCS): A rare debilitating syndrome in which a wide range of respiratory, muscular, neurological, and other symptoms seem to occur with low-level chemical exposure. The causes—and even the existence—of MCS remain controversial.

Off-gassing: The process in which gaseous pollutants are released from products into the environment. This generally applies to volatile organic compounds (VOCs) found in paint, some plastics, cleaning products, PVC flooring, carpeting, particleboard, and other household products and materials.

Organic chemicals: Compounds synthesized from hydrogen and carbon that form the foundation of most modern, man-made chemicals such as plastics, solvents, flame retardants, and many other synthetic substances.

Organic food: The label "organic" is now regulated by the FDA and generally requires that crops are grown and processed without conventional pesticides, artificial fertilizers, or chemical additives. Organically raised animals must be fed organic feed, free of antibiotics and hormones, and comply with certain sustainable farming practices.

PBT chemicals: Chemicals that combine the three insidious traits of *persistence, bioaccumulation,* and *toxicity.* These tend to enter the food web and get biomagnified in the bodies of animals higher up the food chain (including humans).

Persistent chemicals: Because these chemicals don't readily break down in the environment, they tend to linger for years and may spread widely throughout the environment. If continually released, environmental concentrations will also increase over time.

Persistent organic pollutants (POPs): These chemicals, which exhibit the three criteria of PBTs, remain in the environment for many years, become widely distributed geographically, and accumulate in living organisms. POPs include many pesticides, industrial chemicals, and the by-products of industrial processes, such as dioxin (see the "Dirty Dozen" list, page 147).

POPs Convention: See *Stockholm Convention on Persistent Organic Pollutants.*

Right-to-know: The principle that manufacturers and regulators should make information on the toxicity of chemicals readily available to the public.

Stockholm Convention on Persistent Organic Pollutants (POPs): A UN-sponsored international agreement of over 140 countries to ban or greatly restrict the use of 12 of the most dangerous and widespread POPs—and, over time, to add others to the list that meet their criteria.

Testicular dysgenesis syndrome (TDS): A cluster of male sexual development symptoms thought to be linked to environmental chemicals. Symptoms include abnormal development of the sex organs in utero, and low sperm counts, infertility, and testicular germ-cell cancer in adults.

Toxic body burden: The amount of toxic chemicals that are present in the body at any given time. This includes both bioaccumulative chemicals that tend to stay in the body and more easily metabolized chemicals introduced from recent or daily exposures.

Volatile organic compounds (VOCs): These compounds, such as solvents, readily vaporize and enter the air at room temperature. If toxic, they will contribute to indoor air pollution and may pose a health risk. Paints, cleaning products, glues, PVC flooring, and particleboard all commonly contain VOCs. See also *Off-gassing*.

Common Acronyms

BFRs	Brominated flame retardant
BPA or BpA	Bisphenol A
BPT	Bioaccumulative, persistent, and toxic
CPSC	Consumer Products Safety Commission
DDT	Dichloro-diphenyl-trichloroethane
Deca BDE	Deca-brominated diphenyl ether
DEHP	Di(2-ethylhexyl) phthalate
DES	Diethylstilbestrol
EDC	Endocrine-disrupting chemical
EPA	Environmental Protection Agency
FDA	Food and Drug Administration
GNP	Gross national product
MCS	Multiple chemical sensitivity
MDF	Medium-density fiberboard
MIT	Methylisothiazolinone
Octa BDE	Octa-brominated diphenyl ether
PAH	Polycyclic aromatic hydrocarbons
PBDE	Poly-brominated diphenyl ether
PBT	Persistent, bioaccumulative, and toxic

PCB	Polychlorinated biphenyl
Penta BDE	Penta-brominated diphenyl ether
PERC	Perchloroethylene
PFC	Perfluorinated chemicals
PFOA	Perfluorooctanoic acid
PFOS	Perfluorooctane sulfonate
POP	Persistent organic pollutant
PVC	Polyvinyl chloride
REACH	Regulation, Evaluation and Authorisation of Chemicals
RTK	Right-to-know
SLS	Sodium lauryl sulphate
TBT	Tributyltin
TDS	Testicular dysgenesis syndrome
TSCA	Toxic Substances Control Act
VOC	Volatile organic compound
VPVB	Very persistent, very bioaccumulative

The Dirty Dozen

The commercial use of these 12 highly toxic chemicals, found throughout the world, has been banned or severely restricted in over 140 countries under the UN Stockholm Convention on Persistent Organic Pollutants (POPs).

Aldrin—A pesticide applied to soils to kill termites, grasshoppers, corn rootworm, and other insect pests.

Chlordane—Used extensively to control termites and as a broad-spectrum insecticide on a range of agricultural crops.

DDT—Perhaps the best known of the POPs, DDT was widely used during World War II to protect soldiers and civilians from malaria, typhus, and other diseases spread by insects. It continues to be applied against mosquitoes in several countries to control malaria.

Dieldrin—Used principally to control termites and textile pests, dieldrin has also been used to control insect-borne diseases and insects living in agricultural soils.

Dioxins—These chemicals are produced unintentionally due to incomplete combustion, as well as during the manufacture of certain pesticides and other chemicals. In addition, certain kinds of metal recycling and pulp and paper bleaching can release dioxins. Dioxins have also been found in automobile exhaust, tobacco smoke, and wood and coal smoke.

Endrin—This insecticide is sprayed on the leaves of crops such as cotton and grains. It is also used to control mice, voles, and other rodents.

Furans—These compounds are produced unintentionally from the same processes that release dioxins, and they are also found in commercial mixtures of PCBs.

Heptachlor—Primarily employed to kill soil insects and termites, heptachlor has also been used more widely to kill cotton insects, grasshoppers, other crop pests, and malaria-carrying mosquitoes.

Hexachlorobenzene (HCB)—HCB kills fungi that affect food crops. It is also released as a by-product during the manufacture of certain chemicals and as a result of the processes that give rise to dioxins and furans.

Mirex—This insecticide is applied mainly to combat fire ants and other types of ants and termites. It has also been used as a fire retardant in plastics, rubber, and electrical goods.

Polychlorinated Biphenyls (PCBs)—These compounds are employed in industry as heat-exchange fluids, in electric transformers and capacitors, and as additives in paint, carbonless copy paper, sealants, and plastics.

Toxaphene—This insecticide, also called camphechlor, is applied to cotton, cereal grains, fruits, nuts, and vegetables. It has also been used to control ticks and mites in livestock.

Source: Stockholm Convention on Persistent Organic Pollutants (www.pops.int)

Resources

Organizations

Beyond Pesticides: www.beyondpesticides.org

The Center for Health, Environment and Justice: www.chej.org

The Children's Environmental Health Coalition: www.checnet.org

The Collaborative on Health and the Environment: www.healthand
environment.org

Environmental Defense: www.environmentaldefense.org

Environmental Working Group: www.ewg.org

Healthy House Institute: www.healthyhouseinstitute.com

Home Ventilating Institute: www.hvi.org

The National Pesticide Information Center: www.npic.orst.edu

Natural Resources Defense Council: www.nrdc.org

Organic Consumers Association: www.organicconsumers.org

Pesticide Action Network of North America: www.panna.org

Government Agencies

Consumer Products Safety Commission: www.cpsc.gov

Environmental Protection Agency: www.epa.gov

Federal Drug and Food Administration: www.fda.gov

The National Institute of Environmental Health Sciences (a division of
NIH): www.niehs.nih.gov

Safety and Health: www.cdc.gov, www.cdc.gov/niosh

U.S. Centers for Disease Control/National Institute for Occupational

World Heath Organization: www.who.int

Books

Clean and Green—The Complete Guide to Non-Toxic and Environmentally Safe Housekeeping. Annie Berthold Bond (Ceres Press, 1994).

The Healthy House, 4th ed. John Bower (Healthy House Institute, 2000).

Healthy House Building. John Bower (Healthy House Institute, 1997).

Our Stolen Future: Are We Threatening Our Fertility, Intelligence and Survival?—A Scientific Detective Story. Theo Colborn et al. (Plume, 1997). www.ourstolenfuture.org

Publications

Challenged Conceptions: Environmental Chemicals and Fertility. Report published by Women's Health @ Stanford and the Collaborative on Health and the Environment. Free download at: http://obgyn-nw.ucsf.edu/docs/Challenged_Conceptions.pdf.

Environmental Building News. Newsletter and related publications published by www.buildinggreen.com.

Toxic Avoidance Tips

1. Ventilate your home and other indoor environments.

2. Dust and vacuum (with a well-sealed unit) your home regularly.

3. Avoid soft plastics.

4. Avoid synthetic fragrances.

5. Streamline your personal-care range of products and choose organic, fragrance-free, petrochemical-free options wherever possible.

6. Don't buy dry-clean-only clothes.

7. Choose natural floorings over synthetic where possible.

8. Avoid products infused with brominated flame retardants.

9. Avoid nonstick cookware.

10. Avoid stain repellents.

11. Avoid easy-iron clothing.

12. Avoid fungicide-treated socks, shoes, or other clothing.

13. Avoid plastic food boxes.

14. Don't microwave in plastic.

15. Become label savvy—know what to look out for and avoid.

16. Be aware of the VOC levels and other chemicals in DIY products, and always heed safety instructions.

17. Use herbal remedies for your pet's flea infestations.

18. Use herbal remedies for head lice infestations in children.

19. Prepare as much of your diet as possible from fresh ingredients to help avoid the plethora of chemicals used in food processing and packaging.

20. Educate yourself and demand greener alternatives.

21. Ask local authorities how they control weeds in parks and on school playing fields.

22. Query the manufacturer or retailer about the chemical content of products you are suspicious about.

23. Discuss the issue of toxic chemicals in consumer products with other people; word of mouth has always been the best form of public relations, and the more people know and talk about these issues, the more pressure ultimately is bought to bear on the regulators and the industry they are supposed to regulate.

Notes

1
Davis, D. L., G. E. Dinse, and D. G. Hoel: "Decreasing Cardiovascular Disease and Increasing Cancer Among Whites in the U.S. from 1973 through 1987." *Journal of the American Medical Association*, Vol. 271, No. 6 (February 9, 1994): 431–437.

2
Janssen, S., G. Solomon, and T. Schettler: "Chemical Contaminants and Human Disease: A Summary of Evidence by CHE, USA." IPCS Global Assessment on the State of the Science of Endocrine Disruptors, WHO, 2002. Linda S. Birnbaum and Suzanne E. Fenton: "Cancer and Developmental Exposure to Endocrine Disruptors." *Environmental Health Perspectives*, Vol. 111, No. 4 (April 2003): 389–394. D. Clapp, G. Howe, and M. Jacobs Lefevre: *Environmental and Occupational Causes of Cancer: A Review of Recent Scientific Literature*. Lowell Center for Sustainable Production, University of Massachusetts, 2005.

3
Skakkebaek, N. E., E. Rajpert-De Meyts, and K. M. Main: "Testicular Dysgenesis Syndrome: An Increasingly Common Developmental Disorder with Environmental Aspects." *Human Reproduction*, Vol. 16, No. 5 (May 2001): 972–978.

4
Birnbaum, Linda S., and Daniele F. Staskal. "Brominated Flame Retardants: Cause for Concern?" *Environmental Health Perspectives*, Vol. 112, No. 1 (January 2004): 9–17.

5
"Mothers' Milk: Record Levels of Toxic Fire Retardants Found in American Mothers' Breast Milk: Health Risks of PBDEs." Environmental Working Group, USA, 2006.

6

SAB (2006) Science Advisory Board review of the EPA's draft risk assessment of potential human health effects associated with PFOA and its salts. May 30, 2006. EPA-SAB-06-006. US EPA, Washington.

OECD 2002 Environment Directorate Joint Meeting of the Chemicals Committee and the Working Party on Chemicals, Pesticides, and Biotechnology. "Cooperation on Existing Chemicals Hazard Assessment of Perfluorooctane Sulfonate (PFOS) and Its Salts." ENV/JM/RD(2002)17/FINAL. Nov 21, 2002.

KemI 2004. Dossier in support for a nomination of PFOS to the UN-ECE LRTAP Protocol and the Stockholm Convention.

7

Compare the Buncefield disaster, Hertfordshire, UK, December 11, 2005—a massive fire at an oil depot left over three million gallons of highly toxic "firewater" that has proved very tricky to dispose of without contaminating the local environment. See, e.g., http://en.wikipedia.org/wiki/2005_Hertfordshire_Oil_Storage_Terminal_fire and http://www.prnewswire.co.uk/cgi/news/release?id=160501 for more information.

8

Hoppin, Jane A., John W. Brock, Barbara J. Davis, and Donna D. Baird: "Reproducibility of Urinary Phthalate Metabolites in First Morning Urine Samples." *Environmental Health Perspectives,* Vol. 110, No. 5 (May 2002): 515–518.

9

Breast cancer: Muñoz-de-Toro, Monica, Caroline M. Markey, Perinaaz R. Wadia, Enrique H. Luque, Beverly S. Rubin, Carlos Sonnenschein, and Ana M. Soto: "Perinatal Exposure to Bisphenol A Alters Peripubertal Mammary Gland Development in Mice." *Endocrinology,* Vol. 146, No. 9 (2005): 4138–4147.

Immune-system defects: Alizadeh, Mohammad, Fusao Ota, Kazuo Hosoi, Makoto Kato, Tohru Sakai, and Mohammed A. Satter: "Altered Allergic Cytokine and Antibody Response in Mice Treated with Bisphenol A." *Journal of Medical Investigation,* Vol. 53 (2006): 70–80.

Immune-system defects: Yoshino, Shin, Kouya Yamaki, Xiaojuan Li, Tao Sai, Rie Yanagisawa, Hirohisa Takano, Shinji Taneda, Hideyuki Hayashi, and Yoki Mori: "Prenatal Exposure to Bisphenol A Up-Regulates Immune Responses, Including T Helper 1 and T Helper 2 Responses, in Mice." *Immunology,* Vol. 112, No. 3 (July 2004): 489–495.

Insulin resistance and diabetes: Alonso-Magdalena, Paloma, Sumiko Morimoto, Cristina Ripoll, Esther Fuentes, and Angel Nadal: "The Estrogenic Effect of Bisphenol A Disrupts the Pancreatic ß-Cell Function *In Vivo* and Induces Insulin Resistance." *Environmental Health Perspectives,* Vol. 114, No. 1 (January 2006): 106–112.

Male reproductive system defects: vom Saal, Frederick S., and Claude Hughes: "An Extensive New Literature Concerning Low-Dose Effects of Bisphenol A Shows the Need for a New Risk Assessment." *Environmental Health Perspectives,* Vol. 113, No. 8 (August 2005): 926–933.

Miscarriage: Sugiura-Ogasawara, Mayumi, Yasuhiko Ozaki, Shin-ichi Sonta, Tsunehisa Makino, and Kaoru Suzumori: "Exposure to Bisphenol A Is Associated with Recurrent Miscarriage." *Human Reproduction,* Vol. 20, No. 8 (2005): 2325–2329.

Obesity: Masuno, Hiroshi, Teruki Kidani, Keizo Sekiya, Kenshi Sakayama, Takahiko Shiosaka, Haruyasu Yamamoto, and Katsuhisa Honda: "Bisphenol A in Combination with Insulin Can Accelerate the Conversion of 3t3-L1 Fibroblasts to Adipocytes." *Journal of Lipid Research,* Vol. 43 (May 2002): 676–684.

Polycystic ovarian disease: Takeuchi, Toru, Osamu Tsutsumi, Yumiko Ikezuki, Yasushi Takai, and Yuji Taketani: "Positive Relationship between Androgen and the Endocrine Disruptor, Bisphenol A, in Normal Women and Women with Ovarian Dysfunction." *Endocrine Journal,* Vol. 51, No. 2 (2004): 165–169.

Index

About the Authors

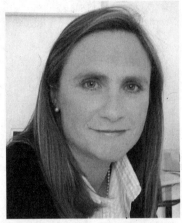 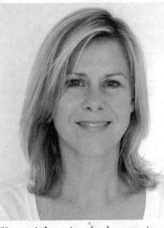

Elizabeth Salter Green is the director of CHEM (Chemicals, Health and Environment Monitoring) Trust, a new organization set up to protect humans and wildlife from harmful chemicals. Prior to her position at CHEM Trust, Elizabeth was director of the WWF-UK Toxics Program for ten years. Her first degree is in physiology, specializing in endocrinology. This was followed by six years of marine research. Her second degree is in international environmental law. While at WWF, Elizabeth was loaned to the UN Balkans Task Force, which studied pollution generated by NATO bombing. Priority work areas for CHEM Trust are endocrine-disrupting chemicals (EDCs), particularly in relation to breast cancer and male reproductive health, and EU chemicals policy and legislation.

Karen Ashton is a freelance writer and arts consultant with a background in PR and advertising. She has always been concerned about environmental issues and first became interested in the subject of toxic chemicals while researching an eco-espionage novel that featured chemical-industry corruption as part of its plot. She is now committed to writing further on the subject for the nonfiction market.